ATLAS OF
LAPAROSCOPIC
TECHNIQUE
FOR GYNECOLOGISTS

ATLAS OF
LAPAROSCOPIC
TECHNIQUE
FOR GYNECOLOGISTS

Edited by *T Tulandi*
MD, FRCS(C), FACOG

Director, Division Reproductive Endocrinology and Infertility
Professor of Obstetrics and Gynecology
McGill University, Royal Victoria Hospital, Montreal, Canada

WB SAUNDERS COMPANY LIMITED
London   Philadelphia   Sydney   Tokyo   Toronto

W. B. Saunders Company Ltd   24–28 Oval Road
London NW1 7DX

The Curtis Center
Independence Square West
Philadelphia, PA 19106-3399, USA

Harcourt Brace & Company
55 Horner Avenue
Toronto, Ontario M8Z 4X6, Canada

Harcourt Brace & Company, Australia
30–52 Smidmore Street
Marrickville, NSW 2204, Australia

Harcourt Brace & Company, Japan, Inc
Ichibancho Central Building, 22-1 Ichibancho
Chiyoda-ku, Tokyo 102, Japan

A catalogue record for this book is available from the British Library

ISBN 0-7020-1914-3

Typeset by Gray Publishing, Tunbridge Wells
Printed in Spain by Printeksa, Bilbao

CONTENTS

LIST OF CONTRIBUTORS

NICHOLAS KADAR
Director of Gynecologic Oncology,
Jersey Shore Medical Center,
Neptune, NJ and Clinical Associate
Professor of Obstetrics and
Gynecology, UMD-Robert Wood
Johnson Medical School, Piscataway,
NJ, U.S.A.

THOMAS L. LYONS
Southeastern Institute for Endoscopic
and Laser Surgery, Atlanta, Georgia,
U.S.A.

PETER MCCOMB
Professor of Obstetrics and
Gynecology, University of British
Columbia, Vancouver, BC, Canada

LISELOTTE METTLER
Professor of Obstetrics and
Gynecology, Klinikum der Christian-
Albrechts-Universität Zu Kiel, Kiel,
Germany

DAVID B. REDWINE
Director, Endometriosis Institute of
Oregon, Bend, Oregon, U.S.A.

HARRY REICH
Wyoming Valley GYN Associates,
Kingston, PA and Community
Hospital of Dobbs Ferry, Dobbs Ferry,
NY, U.S.A.

KURT SEMM
Professor of Obstetrics and
Gynecology, Klinikum der Christian-
Albrechts-Universität Zu Kiel, Kiel,
Germany

HOWARD C. TOPEL
Lutheran General Hospital, Park
Ridge, IL, U.S.A.

TOGAS TULANDI
Professor of Obstetrics and
Gynecology and Director, Division of
Reproductive Endocrinology and
Infertility, McGill University,
Montreal, Quebec, Canada

PREFACE

Many procedures that previously required a laparotomy are now done by laparoscopy. The advantages of laparoscopy are obvious, but for many surgeons a laparoscopic procedure has the disadvantage of taking more time to perform than its laparotomy counterpart. After assisting many gynecologists to perform laparoscopic surgery, it has become apparent that many of them would appreciate guidance on how to make the procedure more efficient and quicker. The purpose of this book is to provide such instruction in a concise, practical, step-by-step illustrated guide on how to perform a range of surgical interventions by laparoscopy. The contributors are surgeons who have many years of experience in the procedures they describe and they offer some simple tips to facilitate the conduct of surgery; it is recognized that with time and experience, each surgeon will then develop his or her own technique.

This is a book for student surgeons, residents, fellows and practising gynecologists who are familiar with laparoscopy for diagnostic purposes or for sterilization. Those who are already performing advanced laparoscopy may also find some tips in this book helpful. Most of the procedures described are done using laparoscopic scissors or electrocautery. The use of a laser as an alternative modality to electrocautery and scissors is also discussed briefly. This book focuses on surgical techniques; the indication for a particular surgical intervention is left to the reader's discretion.

The author is grateful to the contributors, to Brenda Kennedy for her illustrations and to Margaret Macdonald at W. B. Saunders Company Limited for her continuous support and expertise in publishing medical works.

Togas Tulandi M.D.

1 BASIC PRINCIPLES OF LAPAROSCOPIC SURGERY

Togas Tulandi

Advances in technology including instrumentation and video-imaging have led to rapid progress in laparoscopic surgery. Accordingly, many procedures that previously required a laparotomy can be performed by laparoscopy. Operative laparoscopy, however, demands a higher degree of technical skills and a greater variety of equipment than for diagnostic laparoscopy or tubal sterilization. Knowledge of anatomy and pathology and the familiarity of the surgeon with the instruments are mandatory. Depending upon the surgeon's preference, the procedure can be done with either laser, electrocautery or scissors.

SETUP

The setup should ideally involve two video monitors. The monitors are placed on each side of an instrument table which is installed at the end of the operating table between the patient's legs. The surgeon stands facing one monitor on the opposite side and the assistant faces the second monitor. For one video monitor setup, the monitor is placed at the end of an operating table between the patient's legs for easy viewing by both the surgeon and the assistant. A surgical team that is familiar with operative laparoscopy is invaluable. They are responsible for the operation of monopolar or bipolar electrosurgical generators, laser and suction irrigator. They should be knowledgeable of all laparoscopic instruments and

should know how to find a back-up instrument at short notice.

POSITIONING AND PREPARATION

Under low lithotomy position, the patient is placed horizontally until insertion of the laparoscope into the abdominal cavity. Using Allen stirrups or knee braces, the thighs are placed almost parallel to the abdomen (Fig. 1.1). This will facilitate manipulation of instruments. The lateral aspect of the knee should be well padded to prevent peroneal nerve compression. A rigid intrauterine cannula is inserted into the uterus to allow manipulation of the uterus and to permit chromopertubation. I prefer a disposable plastic intrauterine cannula. An intravenous line is inserted through the patient's arm on the assistant's side, and the arm on the side of the operating surgeon should be placed by the patient's side and protected with an ulnar pad. An extended arm will interfere with the surgeon's mobility. Furthermore, brachial plexus neuropathy has been reported after laparoscopic surgery using the steep Trendelenburg position with shoulder braces and the patient's arm extended at 90°. To ascertain that the bladder is empty throughout the procedure, an indwelling catheter is placed inside the bladder and is removed at the end of the operation. When severe adhesion or advanced endometriosis requiring

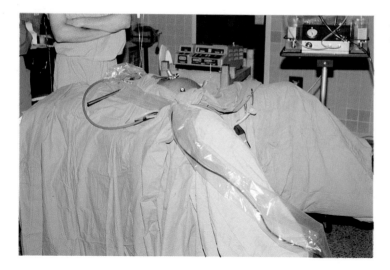

Figure 1.1 *The thighs are placed almost parallel to the abdomen. This will facilitate manipulation of the laparoscopic instruments.*

extensive dissection in the vicinity of the large bowel is suspected, a bowel prep is indicated. Shaving of the abdomen and pubic area is not required. Laparoscopy of the pelvic organs is done in the Trendelenburg position (about 30°).

TROCAR INSERTION

The primary trocar is inserted via a 10-mm infra-umbilical incision. Direct trocar insertion without the use of a Veress needle can be safely done using a disposable trocar. It has a retractable inner trocar and its tip is always sharp. In non-obese women, a Veress needle or primary trocar is inserted at 45° from the horizontal. The aortic bifurcation in non-obese women is located about 4 mm cranial to the umbilicus. In obese women because the bifurcation is approximately 25 mm cranial to the umbilicus, the angle of insertion can be safely increased. In patients who have undergone multiple laparotomies an open laparoscopy using a blunt trocar is recommended. Pneumoperitoneum is achieved by insufflating the abdominal cavity with carbon dioxide (CO_2) gas. The gas is infused at a rate of 1–3 l/min and the intra-abdominal pressure should be below 20 mmHg. The abdomen is observed for global distension and the disappearance of liver dullness. Adequate pneumoperitoneum is usually obtained with 2–3 l of CO_2. After

insertion of the laparoscope, the abdominal cavity should be first evaluated for possible inadvertent injury by the Veress needle or trocar.

I routinely use two to three 5-mm trocars. These trocars are inserted just above the pubic hairline, lateral to the deep epigastric vessels or on the midline (Fig. 1.2). If removal of a specimen via the trocar is anticipated one of the lateral trocars should be at least 10 mm. The trocars should always be inserted under direct laparoscopy control. I use my forefinger as a guard to prevent too deep insertion.

An incisional hernia may occur if the incision is ≥10 mm. A deep suture with 2–0 polyglycolic acid suture to approximate the fascia is required. This is particularly needed for a non-midline incision.

UNDERWATER INSPECTION

Near the completion of each laparoscopic procedure irrigation of the pelvic cavity should be performed and complete haemostasis is mandatory (Fig. 1.3). It should be noted that the pneumoperitoneum acts as a temporary tamponade and the bleeding may occur after the gas is evacuated from the abdominal cavity. Inspection of the operative field after instillation of approximately 500–1000 ml of Ringer's lactate ("examination underwater") allows identification of bleeding points. In a rat model the instillation of a

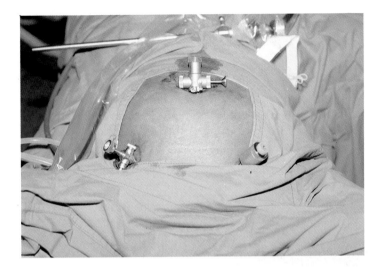

Figure 1.2 *Trocar sites.*

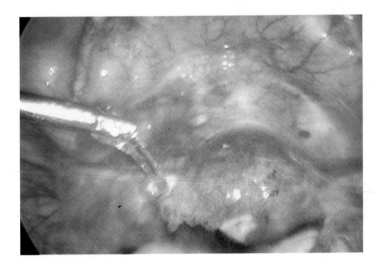

Figure 1.3 *Instillation of Ringer's lactate solution.*

large amount of Ringer's lactate prevents adhesion formation.

ANAESTHESIA

For operative laparoscopy general anaesthesia with endotracheal intubation is mandatory. Assisting ventilation by mask before intubation may inflate the stomach and should be avoided. Otherwise, a nasogastric tube should be inserted to deflate the stomach before insertion of a Veress needle or a trocar. Shoulder braces may be needed for the deep Trendelenburg position. Adequate ventilation is essential during the laparoscopic procedure. Rapid absorption of the CO_2 gas and decrease of lung expansion due to the pneumoperitoneum and Trendelenburg position may result in hypercarbia. Cardiac arrhythmias may then occur.

COMPLICATIONS AND PREVENTION OF INJURY TO DEEP EPIGASTRIC VESSELS

Injury to the deep epigastric vessels is avoided by transilluminating the abdominal wall before trocar insertion and by visualization of the vessels on the peritoneal surface of the anterior abdomen by the laparoscope. The vessels which are located lateral to the obliterated umbilical artery should be avoided (Figs 1.4 and 1.5). Despite these measures occasionally a large vessel is injured and brisk bleeding occurs. This can be controlled by a figure-of-eight suture with a retention suture. Under direct laparoscopy control, a large needle through the whole thickness of the abdominal wall is placed with the trocar *in situ*. The trocar is then removed and the suture is tied. Another alternative is by using a Foley catheter. A #16 catheter is first inserted into the abdominal cavity via the trocar. The balloon is inflated, the trocar is removed and the catheter is pulled outside until the balloon is tightly compressing the bleeding site. A clamp is placed on the outer side of the catheter at the skin level to maintain traction and haemostasis. The suture or the catheter can be removed in 24 hours.

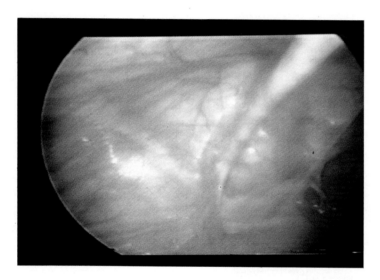

Figure 1.4 *Deep epigastric vessels (left) are located lateral to the obliterated umbilical artery (centre).*

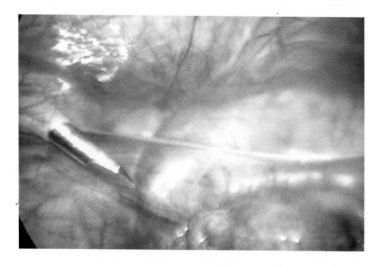

Figure 1.5 *Secondary trocar should be inserted under laparoscopic control lateral to the deep epigastric vessels.*

SUGGESTED READING

Hurd WH, Bude RO, DeLancey JOL, Pearl ML: The relationship of the umbilicus to the aortic bifurcation: Implications for laparoscopic technique. *Obstet Gynecol* 1992 **80**:48–51.

Pagidas K, Tulandi T: Effects of Ringer's lactate, INTERCEED(TC7) and Gore-Tex surgical membrane on postsurgical adhesion formation. *Fertil Steril* 1992 **57**:199–201.

Reich H: New laparoscopic techniques. In Sutton C and Diamond MP (eds) *Endoscopic Surgery for Gynaecologists*. WB Saunders, London, 1993, pp. 28–39.

Tulandi T: Clinical results of laser and electro-diathermy. In Sutton C and Diamond MP (eds) *Endoscopic Surgery for Gynaecologists*. WB Saunders, London, 1993, pp. 84–89.

2 INSTRUMENTATION

Togas Tulandi

Operative laparoscopy cannot be carried out adequately using the standard diagnostic laparoscopy or tubal sterilization equipment. More equipment and a greater variety of instruments are needed. This chapter will discuss basic operative laparoscopic instrumentation. Equipment that is already available for diagnostic laparoscopy or sterilization will not be discussed. New instruments are being continuously developed and tested, and some of them may replace the existing instruments. It is crucial to have a good knowledge of the instruments. This will facilitate the conduct of surgery, and ensure that the instruments are used wisely so that they will last longer. More importantly, a thorough knowledge of the instruments increases the safety of laparoscopic surgery. Beginners tend to purchase a wide variety of instruments that may or may not be eventually used. It is better to start with instruments described in this chapter and then the set can be gradually expanded with instruments of your choice. The availability of good and well-maintained laparoscopic instruments is invaluable. Back-up instruments are mandatory and may be required at short notice.

LAPAROSCOPE

A 10-mm straightforward 0° laparoscope has a large viewing angle. It is the best laparoscope for diagnostic as well as for operative surgery. A laparoscope with a laser channel is an alternative.

TROCARS AND REDUCER

Two trocars of 10 mm diameter and two or three trocars of 5 mm should be available. The secondary trocars are usually 5 mm, but one of them should be 12 mm if removal of a specimen is anticipated. Here, a reduction sleeve (reducer) with 5 mm diameter is necessary (Fig. 2.1). An ultrashort reduction sleeve (37.5 mm length) is also available. The length of the trocar is usually 105 mm. Depending upon the abdominal thickness, shorter trocars (50 mm) that allow freer access to the pelvic structures can be used. Some trocars have spiral threads on the outside. The threads

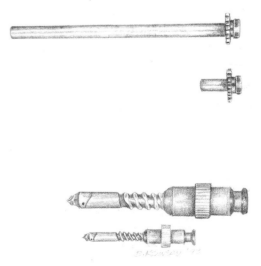

Figure 2.1 *Reduction sleeve and short trocars with spiral threads.*

prevent slippage of the trocar during removal of ancillary instruments such as forceps or scissors. It is desirable to have secondary trocars without valves. The valves interfere with insertion and removal of ancillary instruments, specimen or suture materials. Non-disposable trocars are more economical, but their sharpness should be maintained; otherwise, disposable trocars should be used. For open laparoscopy a blunt tip trocar is required.

CAMERA AND MONITOR

These are mandatory for the safe conduct of operative laparoscopy. Maximum image quality can be obtained with the use of three-chip technology, high-intensity light (such as xenon or halogen bulbs) and a high-resolution video monitor. A beamsplitter on the camera head for simultaneous viewing by endoscope and monitor decreases the amount of light and is not necessary. Surgery can be done safely without looking into the laparoscope. A video-recorder to record the surgery can be utilized for documentation and teaching. A mobile storage video-cart for the monitor, light source, insufflator, video-recorder or video-printer protects this expensive equipment from premature wear and tear and from accidents.

HIGH-FLOW INSUFFLATOR

Frequent instrument changes and constant irrigation and aspiration during a procedure lead to a rapid loss of pneumoperitoneum. To maintain pneumoperitoneum, a high-flow insufflator that administers up to 10 l of gas per minute is a prerequisite.

SUCTION IRRIGATOR

A powerful irrigation pump that can deliver pressure of up to 800 mmHg is invaluable for operative laparoscopy. An example is the Nezhat–Dorsey suction irrigation system. It is an efficient irrigator and it helps to obtain an accurate haemostasis. It can also be used to separate tissue planes, adhesions, ovarian

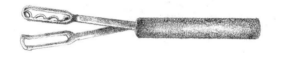

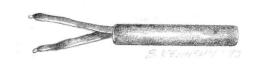

Figure 2.2 *Bipolar grasping forceps and microforceps.*

cyst wall or to flush products of conception from the Fallopian tube.

BIPOLAR AND UNIPOLAR INSTRUMENTS

Bipolar grasping forceps should always be readily available for haemostasis (Fig. 2.2). These are not replaceable by unipolar forceps or a laser. A 5-mm bipolar microforceps allows accurate coagulation. Among unipolar instruments my favourites are unipolar scissors and a 1-mm needle electrode that can be inserted into a built-in channel suction irrigator (Fig. 2.3).

DISSECTING AND GRASPING FORCEPS

There are two types of grasping forceps: traumatic or atraumatic forceps (Fig. 2.4). I usually use the 5-mm SEMM atraumatic grasping forceps and a Babcock clamp. For secure grasping, 5-mm grasping forceps with 2×2 teeth can be used. A 10-mm claw forceps is useful for specimen removal (ovarian cyst, ovary, myoma, etc.) via a 12-mm secondary trocar. Due to its powerful and sharp jaws, this forceps must only be applied to the tissue to be removed.

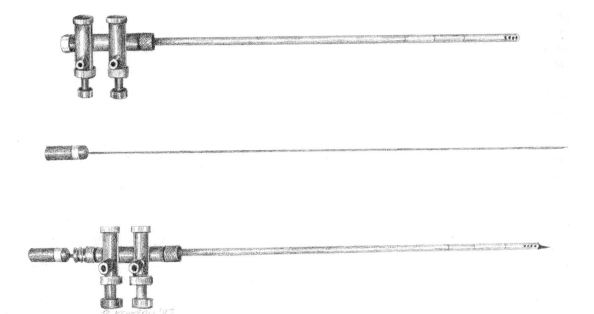

Figure 2.3 *Suction irrigator: a unipolar needle electrode can be incorporated into the system.*

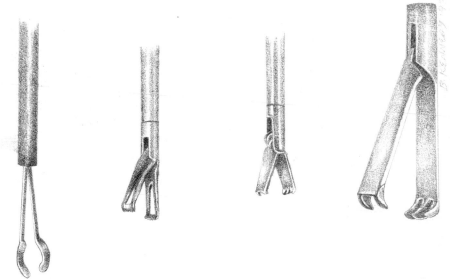

Figure 2.4 *Atraumatic grasping forceps, Babcock forceps, grasping forceps with teeth, 10-mm claw forceps.*

SCISSORS

Cold instruments including scissors remain the best tools for dissection in reproductive surgery. A wide variety of scissors are available. The most commonly used scissors are shown in Fig. 2.5. It is important to have scissors that cut and do not tear the tissue. A combination of cutting and coagulating can be obtained by incorporating electrical energy into the scissors. An example is the unipolar Metzenbaum scissors. Because scissors tend to become dull, frequent sharpening is necessary. Other types of scissors including hook scissors and microdissecting scissors should also be available.

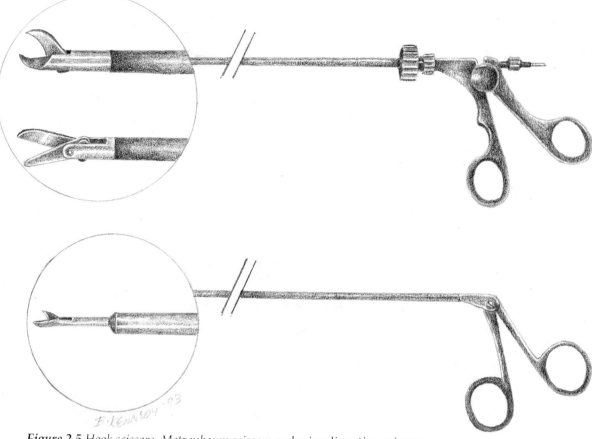

Figure 2.5 *Hook scissors, Metzenbaum scissors and microdissecting scissors.*

SUTURE AND LIGATURE

Needle holders and suture forceps for a straight or ski needle and for a curved needle should be available (Fig. 2.6). The use of a knot pusher (suture manipulator) allows extracorporeal tying and facilitates the procedure. I find that the use of a non-disposable knot pusher with a fenestration at the end (Fig. 2.6) markedly expedites the process of knot tying. After suturing, the needle is extracted outside the abdominal cavity and inserted into the fenestration. The surgeon makes a knot and the knot is then pushed into the abdominal cavity. The procedure is repeated several times. Other types of knot pusher that do not have a fenestration require the surgeon to place the suture in the groove of the knot pusher. This takes time especially in a darkened operating theatre. The availability of a pretied ligature (Endoloops,

Rx Ethicon Inc., Sommerville, NJ; PercLoop, Laparomed, Irvine, CA) permits easy ligature of structures including appendix, Fallopian tube or ovary.

MISCELLANEOUS

Administration of a dilute solution of vasopressin decreases bleeding from the site of tubal anastomosis, ectopic pregnancy or myomectomy. A spinal needle can be used, but it is not rigid and bends easily. A non-disposable injection needle (shaft diameter of 5 mm) (Fig. 2.7) that can be inserted via a secondary trocar is a better instrument. Stabilizing a myoma during dissection and enucleation can be accomplished using a 5-mm corkscrew. Occasionally, a morcellator is needed to break large specimens such as myoma into small pieces and to remove

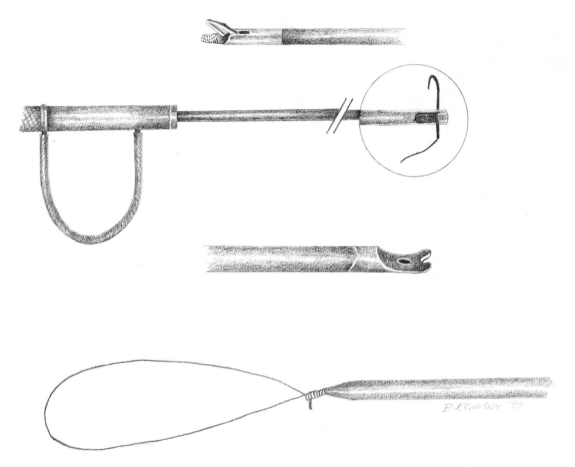

Figure 2.6 *Needle holder for a straight or ski needle, needle holder for a curved needle, suture manipulator (knot pusher) with a fenestration and pretied ligature (loop).*

them. A clip and staple applicator may be needed, although they are not essential.

LASER

Laser, electrocautery or regular scissors are merely surgical modalities. The clinical results depend more on the surgeon's experience and preference and proper patient selection than the type of surgical modality used. The use of a laser via a built-in channel of the laparoscope liberates one of the secondary trocars which can be replaced by another ancillary instrument.

DISPOSABLE INSTRUMENTS

There are many disposable instruments available. For economical reasons, I use mainly non-disposable instruments; disposable instruments are utilized when necessary. However, it is recommended to have some disposable instruments in the operating theatre as a back-up.

BASIC INSTRUMENTS

This is a list of the basic instruments. Back-up instruments are desirable.

1. A 10-mm straightforward laparoscope 0°.
2. Trocars:
   (a) 10-mm primary trocar,
   (b) 12-mm secondary trocar,
   (c) 5-mm secondary trocars (at least three).

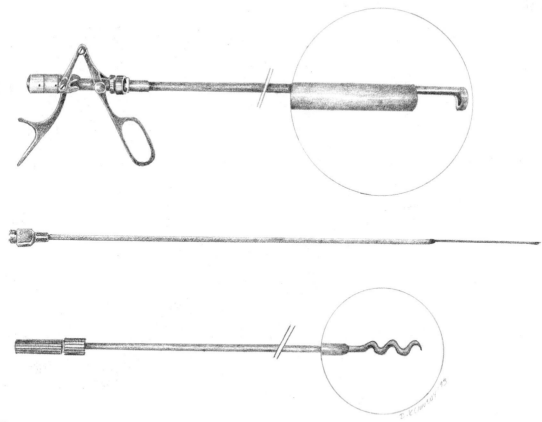

Figure 2.7 *Morcellator, injection needle and myoma screw.*

3. A 5-mm reduction sleeve.
4. Suction irrigation system.
5. Bipolar forceps with cable:
   (a) bipolar grasping forceps,
   (b) bipolar microforceps.
6. Unipolar instruments with cable:
   (a) 1-mm needle electrode,
   (b) unipolar scissors.
7. Forceps:
   (a) SEMM atraumatic grasping forceps,
   (b) Babcock forceps,
   (c) 5-mm grasping forceps with 2 × 2 teeth,
   (d) 10-mm claw forceps.
8. Scissors:
   (a) Metzenbaum rotating forceps,
   (b) hook scissors,
   (c) microdissecting scissors.
9. Suture and ligature:
   (a) needle holder for a straight or ski needle,
   (b) needle holder for a curved needle,
   (c) suture manipulator (knot pusher).
10. Miscellaneous:
    (a) 5-mm injection needle,
    (b) myoma corkscrew,
    (c) morcellator,
    (d) pretied ligature.

SUGGESTED READING

Hasson HM: Open laparoscopy: A report of 150 cases. *J Reprod Med* 1974 **12**:234–238.

Reich H: New laparoscopic techniques. In Sutton C and Diamond MP (eds) *Endoscopic Surgery for Gynaecologists*. WB Saunders, London, 1993, pp. 28–39.

Tulandi T: Clinical results of laser and electrodiathermy. In Sutton C and Diamond MP (eds) *Endoscopic Surgery for Gynaecologists*. WB Saunders, London, 1993, pp. 84–89.

3 LAPAROSCOPIC SUTURING: MICROSUTURING AND EXTRACORPOREAL TYING

Peter McComb

The ability to place sutures by laparoscopy has facilitated procedures such as oophorectomy, salpingectomy and adnexectomy. For these procedures the suture sizes have been 4–0 or heavier. These large suture sizes have limitations for reproductive surgery. As a residual foreign body, they may induce adhesion formation.

Laparoscopic surgery can fulfil the prerequisites of basic principles of microsurgery including constant temperature and humidity, reduced peritoneal injury, magnification, and when performed carefully, gentle tissue handling. Thus, the ability to use a microsuture of size 6–0 or less completes the prerequisites for a true "microsurgical approach" by laparoscopy.

The distinct advantage of the technique is the extracorporeal tying of the knot. Attempts to knot-tie microsuture within the peritoneal cavity are hampered by the abdominal wall, because it acts as a fulcrum for each of the instruments. The surgeon is forced to use the short end of the lever to create motion at its long end; a disadvantage when the aim is to achieve small precise movements at the long end of the lever. Also, intracorporeal knot formation with microsuture is made difficult by the attraction of the suture to peritoneal surfaces by fluid surface tension.

A particular form of knot pusher is required. It is a 300 mm long, partly hollow plastic tube with a single fenestration 1 mm from the open end of the tubing or a non-disposable metal knot pusher as described in Chapter 2.

SUTURING TECHNIQUE

1. The needle and suture are introduced into the peritoneal cavity with a 3-mm diameter needle driver grasping the suture approximately 10 mm from the needle (Fig. 3.1). Once in the pelvic cavity, the suture and needle are detached from the needle driver by placing it on the uterine serosa. The surface tension of the peritoneal fluid retains the needle. It is then picked up in the jaws of the driver.

2. The needle is passed through the tissues. The needle is then drawn from the peritoneal cavity through the 3-mm reduction sleeve (the cannula for introduction of the suture) with the needle driver (Fig. 3.2).

3. The throws of the knot are completed extracorporeally. After each throw, one end of the suture is threaded into the open end of the knot pusher and out of the fenestration. The other end of the suture remains free (Fig. 3.3).

4. Equal tension is next applied to both ends of the suture, and the knot is slid down the length of the suture to apply it to the tissue (Fig. 3.4). This process is repeated to complete a surgical knot. The suture is cut with scissors and the loose suture ends are withdrawn. With experience, each suture takes only a few minutes to place.

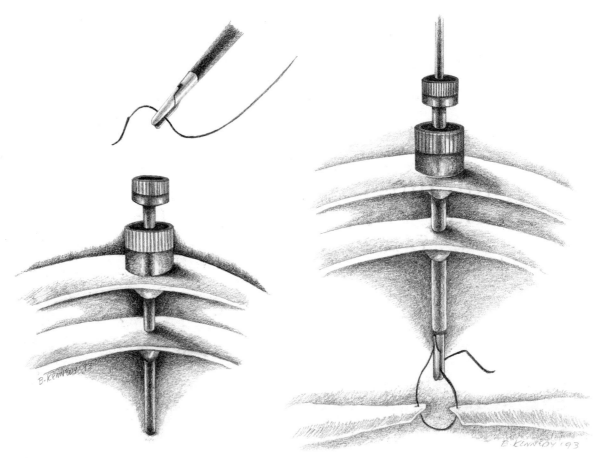

Figure 3.1 The needle is introduced into the peritoneal cavity by grasping the suture approximately 10 mm from the needle.

Figure 3.2 Withdrawing the suture from the peritoneal cavity by grasping the suture as in Fig. 3.1.

POTENTIAL COMPLICATIONS AND THEIR PREVENTION

1. The needle may traumatize a vessel or intestine. The diameter is equal to a 30-gauge needle and is unlikely to require anything more than pressure on the vessel, or close examination of the bowel. This is to ensure that the needle has pierced the bowel cleanly instead of causing a laceration. To avoid these inadvertent injuries, the surgeon must continuously watch the needle when it is mounted in the needle driver.
2. The suture and or needle may be lost. It is rare to lose a needle intra-abdominally. The magnification and illumination afforded by the laparoscope minimize this occurrence. If a needle is lost, radiological localization and use of an intraperitoneal magnetized probe is required.
3. Suture of tissues has a potential to entrap intestine in a ring of tissue. Such a space should be closed.

CONTRAINDICATIONS

There are many reproductive operations that may need microsuture. To date, tubal anastomosis is still best performed by laparotomy than by laparoscopy.

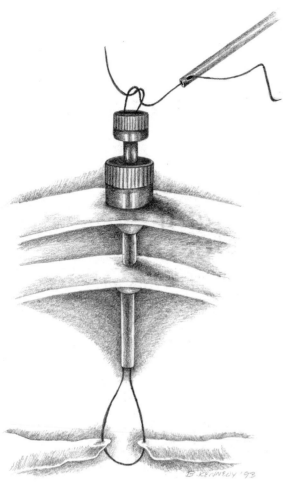

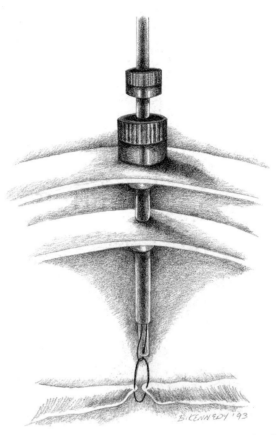

Figure 3.3 *The needle is inserted into the fenestration of the knot pusher before sliding the knot down into the peritoneal cavity.*

Figure 3.4 *Equal tension is applied to both ends of the suture and the knot is tightened with the help of the knot pusher.*

SUGGESTED READING

McComb PF: A new suturing instrument that allows the use of microsuture at laparoscopy. *Fertil Steril* 1992 **57**:936–938.

4 LAPAROSCOPIC SUTURING: INTRACORPOREAL ENDOSUTURING

Howard C. Topel

Endosuturing is a skill necessary for performing a variety of advanced laparoscopic operations. As with conventional open surgery, laparoscopic suturing techniques permit restoration of normal anatomical relationships, organ reconstruction, approximation of tissue planes, and establishment of haemostasis. There are three suturing methods adapted to laparoscopic techniques: endoloop, extracorporeal and intracorporeal.

Once limited to only short straight needles, endosuturing can now be performed with curved needles and a wide variety of suture materials and sizes. Curved needle suturing provides great flexibility and easier adaptation to a two-dimensional video working field. New curved needle drivers have been designed to firmly hold the needle with minimal instability at the tip. This permits curved needles (i.e. SH, CT-3) to be driven through tissue of varying thickness and consistency. In addition, the suture needle can be precisely positioned and passed through tissue with a rotational motion similar to open laparotomy suturing.

A curved needle and suture can be introduced into the abdominal cavity in the following manner:

1. Advance the curved needle driver through the 10 mm suture introducer channel.
2. Grasp the tail end of the suture in the needle driver jaws.
3. Pull the needle driver back through the suture introducer, allowing the suture needle (SH, CT-3) to hang freely beyond the end of the introducer (Fig. 4.1).
4. Release the suture from the jaws of the needle driver.
5. While stabilizing the suture line inside the channel, advance the needle driver back down the introducer.
6. Secure the suture needle (at the needle–suture junction) in the needle driver jaws, keeping the needle curve parallel to the driver and suture introducer.
7. Pull the suture taut (not tight). Then, withdraw the loaded needle driver into the introducer until the entire suture needle is inside the distal end.
8. Cut the excess suture, leaving approximately 25 mm or less exposed at the proximal end of the introducer. The critical suture length is 80–90 mm.
9. The loaded introducer is then re-advanced through the 10/11 mm trocar into the abdominal cavity (Fig. 4.1).
10. Following needle placement into the tissue, the entire length of suture can be brought into the abdominal cavity, and the suture ends can then be equalized in length in preparation for tying.
11. For needle removal, grasp the suture within the jaws of the needle driver 20 mm from the needle. Then cut the suture, and withdraw the needle into the introducer channel (Fig. 4.2).

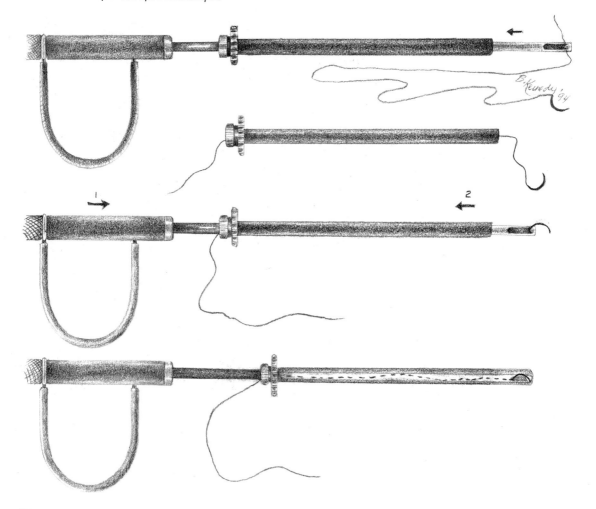

Figure 4.1 *From top to bottom: the end of the suture is grasped with a needle driver and then withdrawn into the introducer until it is completely outside the introducer. The needle holder is reinserted into the introducer (1) and the needle is positioned to allow withdrawal of the loaded needle driver into the introducer (2). This loaded introducer can now be inserted into the abdominal cavity and is ready to be used.*

12. The needle driver, suture needle, and introducer are withdrawn all at once through the trocar port, leaving the trocar in place.
13. The suture is now ready for intra-abdominal knot-tying.

This introduction and retrieval of sutures/needles is designed to control the curved needle at all times, in order to prevent inadvertent tissue injury, or loss of the needle within the abdominal cavity. Intracorporeal knot-tying can be a tedious, time-consuming, and, often, frustrating experience. However,

with patience and a great amount of practice, intra-abdominal knot-tying can be mastered and can be a valuable endoscopic skill. There are two types of intracorporeal knot-tying: classic instrument tie and a new "twist" technique.

The classic instrument knot-tying technique is similar to that performed at laparotomy. However, this classic approach is difficult to perform off of a video monitor, and with finer suture material. A new intracorporeal "twist" knot-tying technique greatly simplifies endoscopic tying. This technique is illustrated in Fig. 4.3. It is applicable to all suture sizes and

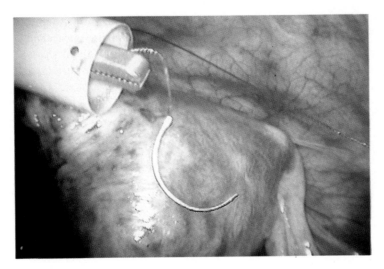

Figure 4.2 *Removal of the needle by grasping the suture with a needle driver approximately 20 mm from the needle and then withdrawing into the introducer.*

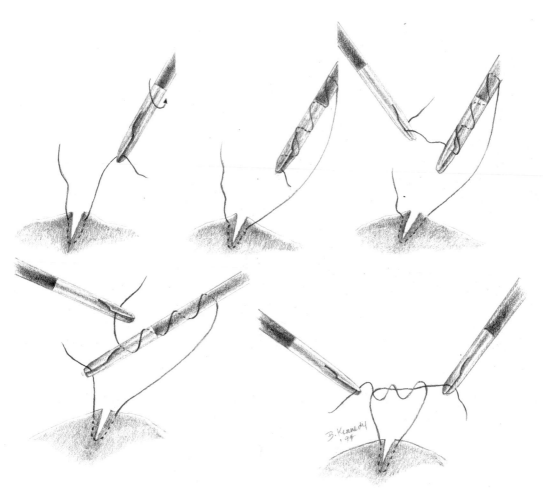

Figure 4.3 *Knot-tying with a "twist" technique.*

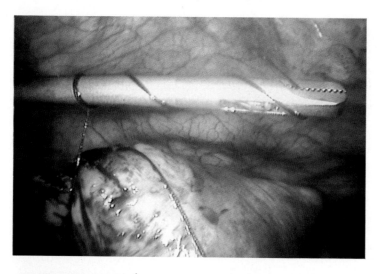

Figure 4.4 *Uterine closure using the "twist" technique: one end of the suture is rotated up the shaft of a grasping instrument until three or four loops are formed.*

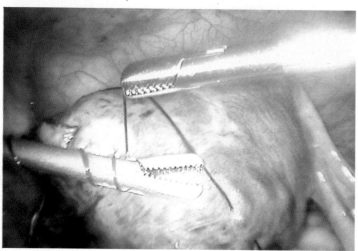

Figure 4.5 *A second grasper removes the suture end from the jaws of the rotating grasper, and slides the end upward along the shaft. The other free suture end is now grasped by the first grasper.*

is designed to consistently form a square double "surgeon" knot with minimal slippage. One end of the suture is rotated up the shaft of a 5-mm grasping instrument until three or four loops are formed (Fig. 4.4). A second grasper removes the suture end from the jaws of the rotating grasper, and slides the end upward along the shaft (Fig. 4.5). The other free suture end is now grasped by the first grasper. As both instruments are pulled in opposite directions, a square double knot is formed (Fig. 4.6). The knot can be tightened against the tissue surface and will not loosen as a second knot is similarly fashioned and positioned onto the tissue.

This "twist" technique provides excellent approximation of heavy tissue under tension, such as with uterine reconstruction following myomectomy. In addition, fine microsurgical knot-tying with delicate suture is readily accomplished with this technique. Often, a suture may be the only method to control bleeding. The "twist" knot-tie is a reliable and consistent way to form a non-slipping knot and establish haemostasis.

Laparoscopic surgery does not preclude the ability to perform continuous endosuturing. With the aid of a specially designed applier (Fig. 4.7), a PDS clip, called a "Laparo-tye", can be attached to the suture end. One clip serves to anchor the start of the suture line, while a second PDS clip secures the

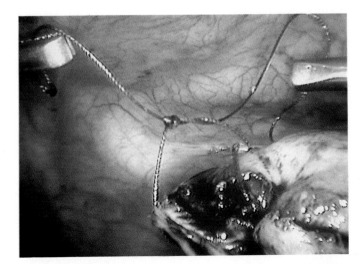

Figure 4.6 *As both instruments are pulled in opposite directions, a square double knot is formed.*

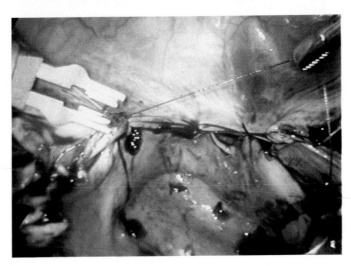

Figure 4.7 *Continuous suturing with the help of a "Laparo-tye" to anchor the beginning of the suture line.*

continuous locking closure. This continuous technique, employing PDS clips, approximates the large uterine defect following myomectomy with an excellent anatomical reconstruction.

With the continuous advancement toward performing more difficult operations, the necessity for improved laparoscopic suturing skills is crucial. Only great patience and hours of dedicated practice will allow the endosurgeon to develop the dexterity and confidence to perform endosuturing. However, once mastered, laparoscopic suturing will permit the successful completion of complex operations with fewer complications, and with an excellent surgical end result.

5 TREATMENT OF ENDOMETRIOSIS

David B. Redwine

Because medical therapy does not eradicate endometriosis, laparoscopic treatment of endometriosis is increasingly popular. Available techniques include electrocoagulation, laser vaporization, and excision using scissors, electrosurgery or laser. Electrocoagulation and laser vaporization risk injury to underlying vascular structures and do not have long-term follow-up validating their efficacy in eradicating or reducing endometriosis. Excision allows safe treatment of invasive disease even over vital structures. Importantly, long-term follow-up is available which strongly suggests efficacy. For these reasons, surgeons are increasingly excising endometriosis.

STAGES IN THE PROCEDURE

Safety considerations

Modern monopolar electrosurgery depends on tissue resistance to electron flow generating tissue heat resulting in vaporization or coagulation tissue. Electrons are delivered to the tissue through an active electrode which may be a scissors, needle, grasper, or any other conducting tool. High current densities are necessary for efficient electrosurgery. Pure cutting current has a constant but smaller peak to peak voltage than does coagulation current and is primarily used when cutting thin tissue like peritoneum. Coagulation current has a higher peak to peak voltage which

is "on" only a fraction of the time. This higher voltage provides more power to push electrons through tissue, making coagulation current useful for cutting retroperitoneal fibrosis or parenchymal structures such as the uterosacral ligaments.

In applying electrosurgical energy to tissue, it is necessary to avoid pillowing of tissue around the tip of the active electrode. Because the greater surface area in contact with tissue will result in a lower current density and increased coagulation effects rather than cutting effects. To avoid undesired pillowing, the electrode is activated before tissue is contacted so cutting begins instantly. The tissue to be cut should be on stretch at all times so that the tissue separates away from the active electrode tip as cutting occurs. The electrode is not always activated, and much of the safety and efficacy of monopolar electrosurgery depends on blunt dissection alternating with brief bursts of electrosurgical cutting when sufficient separation of normal tissue has occurred.

Endometriosis is a disease most commonly found on the peritoneal surface, so excision of involved peritoneum is the fundamental technique used. Whether the surgeon excises endometriosis using scissors, electrosurgery, or laser, an immutable principle of safe surgery is to *separate diseased tissue from normal tissue before application of the surgical energy form*. Most commonly, this is done by grasping the tissue to be removed and drawing it strongly medially, thus elevating the tissue from underlying vital structures before cutting mechanically, electrosurgically, or with laser. This medial traction is also important to avoid pillowing around the active electrode. With fibrotic invasive endometriosis, blunt or sharp dissection with scissors is necessary to separate normal tissue from abnormal tissue before applying the effective surgical energy to the remaining tissue tendrils held on stretch by medial traction.

Endometriosis is a disease of predictable patterns of pelvic involvement, with or without local invasion. Because of this, only a few basic techniques are necessary for successful excision anywhere in the pelvis. These techniques include superficial excision, deep excision, resection of a uterosacral ligament, and ovarian cystectomy. A skilled surgeon can build on these basic techniques to include bowel resection for endometriosis which is covered in Chapter 19.

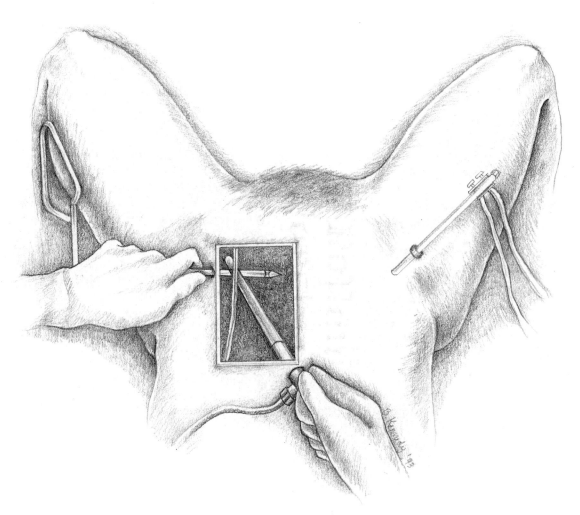

Figure 5.1 *A triple puncture technique is used. After the laparoscope has been inserted through the umbilical incision, it is used to elevate the anterior abdominal wall in the region of the inferior epigastric vessels. A 5.5-mm trocar placed lateral to the inferior epigastric vessels is then passed horizontally beneath the laparoscope into the peritoneal space. This horizontal insertion decreases the likelihood of damage to deeper vascular structures.*

PROCEDURE

I inserted the secondary trocars by elevating the anterior abdominal wall with the laparoscope. Two 5.5-mm trocars are placed in the lower quadrants lateral to the inferior epigastric vessels (Fig. 5.1), one on the right for a suction irrigator, another on the left for an atraumatic grasper. A pair of 3-mm monopolar scissors is passed down the operating channel of the laparoscope and connected to an electrosurgical generator supplying 70 or more watts of pure cutting current and 50 watts of coagulation current controlled by foot pedals.

SUPERFICIAL RESECTION

The abnormal peritoneum is grasped and drawn medially (Fig. 5.2), elevating it away from underlying vital structures. With a "touch cut" using pure cutting current, the active electrode creates a small hole in the adjacent normal peritoneum (Fig. 5.3). The scissors then bluntly undermine the abnormal peritoneum, separating it from the underlying vital structures. With a few strokes using cutting current, the abnormal tissue is excised.

DEEP RESECTION

Some endometriotic lesions are invasive, and retroperitoneal fibrosis can encroach upon or surround vital structures such as the ureter, pelvic vessels or nerves. The principles of resection of deep disease are similar to those

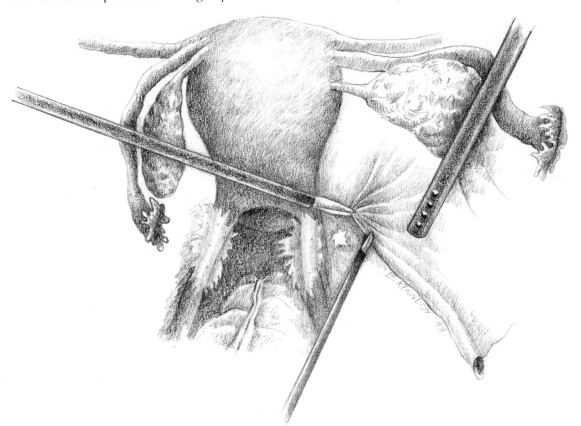

Figure 5.2 *The right tube and ovary are retracted laterally with the suction irrigator. Invasive endometriosis is seen in both uterosacral ligaments. The graspers are elevating the peritoneum adjacent to a superficial lesion of endometriosis. By grasping and elevating the peritoneum away from the underlying vital structures, peritoneal incisions and resections can occur toward the centre of the pelvis away from vital structures of the pelvic sidewall.*

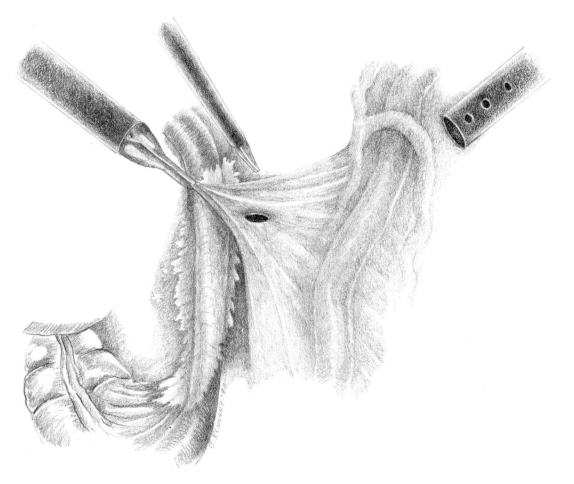

Figure 5.3 *The peritoneum is grasped and pulled away from the right broad ligament. A touch cut has been created with the 3-mm scissors using 70–90 watts of pure cutting current.*

of superficial resections, with two important differences: (1) retroperitoneal blunt dissection is more vigorous and demanding because of the fibrosis; (2) coagulation current is most frequently used retroperitoneally.

Normal peritoneum adjacent to the invasive lesion is entered with a touch cut (Fig. 5.3), then retroperitoneal blunt dissection is used to release normal structures from surrounding fibrosis. This will frequently require ureterolysis or angiolysis. The ureter is a surprisingly resilient structure which will not be injured even by vigorous blunt dissection against it. Usually, the invasive lesion can be grasped and drawn away from the ureter, with the scissors repeatedly pushing into the space between the ureter and the

invasive lesion. This will develop and isolate tendrils of tissue which can then be transected with short bursts of coagulating current. It is sometimes necessary to grasp the ureter firmly and pull on it to achieve counter-traction to advance the dissection. Traction can also be applied to the uterine artery but not to thin-walled veins which may tear.

In the cul de sac, invasive disease may encroach upon the rectum. It is necessary to inspect the cul de sac closely in order to identify the coloration of the colon, which may blend almost imperceptibly with the coloration of normal peritoneum. Just as with ureterolysis, the abnormal tissue is forcibly separated from the rectum with blunt dissection. This can usually be applied tangentially to the bowel wall so the chance of damage to the bowel is minimal. Anteriorly, invasive disease will rarely involve the bladder muscularis.

RESECTION OF THE UTEROSACRAL LIGAMENT

This technique is necessary to remove invasive disease of the uterosacral ligament and does not seem to result in defects of pelvic floor support. It also serves as a foundation for *en bloc* resection of the pelvic floor for treatment of the obliterated cul de sac described in Chapter 19. The key to resection of this ligament is a releasing incision made in normal peritoneum lateral and parallel to the ligament using 70 to 90 watts of cutting current (Figs 5.4 and 5.5). This incision allows the ureter and uterine vessels to separate from the area of the uterosacral ligament (Fig. 5.6), assisted by blunt dissection laterally (Fig. 5.7). A blunt probe can be used to partially undermine the ligament, particularly near its insertion into the posterior cervix. A peritoneal incision is made medial to the ligament and the rectum is identified and bluntly separated from the vicinity of the ligament. The ligament is then amputated at its insertion into the posterior cervix (Fig. 5.8) and shaved off the underlying pelvic floor (Fig. 5.9) using 50 watts of coagulation current. Some patients

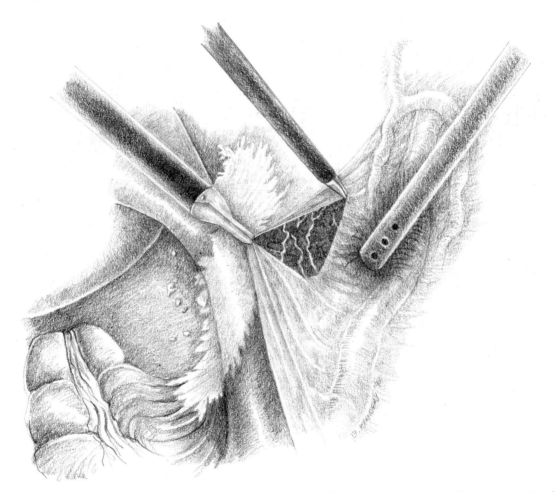

Figure 5.4 *The suction irrigator pulls the ureter laterally. The graspers keep the peritoneum on stretch while the 3-mm monopolar scissors create an electro-surgical peritoneal incision lateral to the right uterosacral ligament. Care is taken to incise only the peritoneum.*

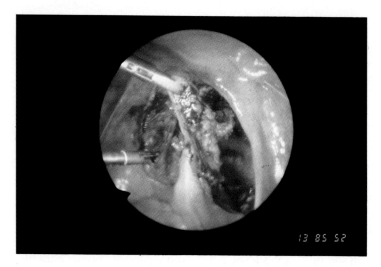

Figure 5.5 *A line of incision has been created in the peritoneum around the left uterosacral ligament, which is involved by white, fibrotic, invasive endometriosis.*

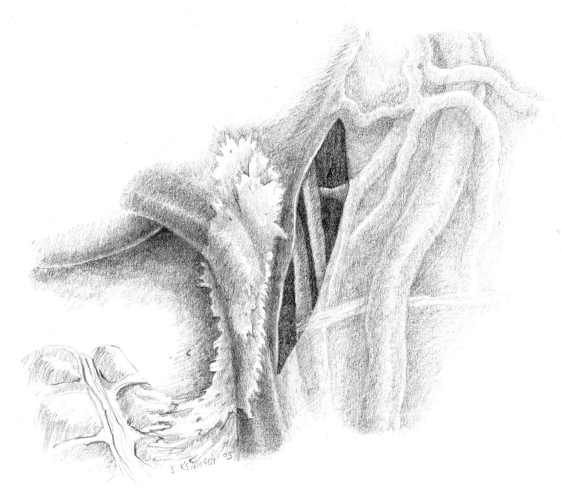

Figure 5.6 *The peritoneal incision has been created lateral and parallel to the right uterosacral ligament. Notice the vessels which course superiorly from the region of the posterior vaginal wall. These vessels are more likely to be damaged at this point than are the uterine vessels or the ureter.*

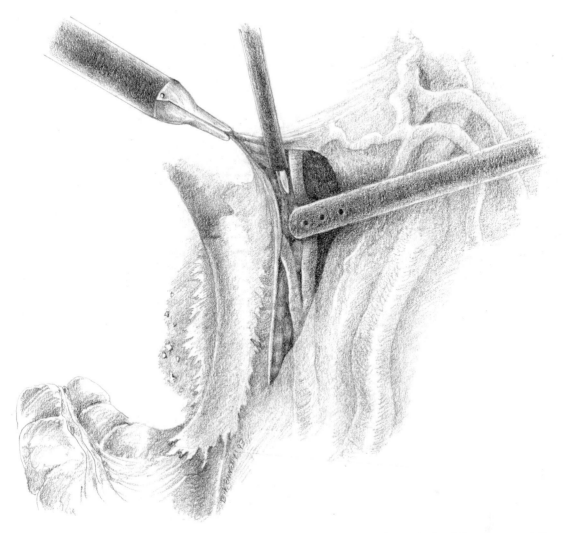

Figure 5.7 *Fibrotic retroperitoneal fibrosis associated with invasive endometriosis of the uterosacral ligament is being dissected off of the vessels ascending from the posterior vaginal wall. This is done with blunt dissection using the 3-mm scissors and counter-traction applied with the suction irrigator and the graspers.*

may require only isolated resection of the involved peritoneum for removal of superficial disease (Figs 5.10 and 5.11), while others may require deep dissection into the sidewall for removal of all invasive disease (Fig. 5.12).

Extensive resection of endometriosis may result in an increased frequency of overnight hospital stays due to nausea and vomiting, although selected patients may leave the afternoon or evening following surgery.

Medical therapy is not necessary for effective treatment of endometriosis. The first two menstrual flows may be unusually painful.

POTENTIAL COMPLICATIONS

If electro-excision is used and the tissue to be cut is not held under strong tension, coagulation instead of cutting will occur. This not only wastes time, but may injure or obscure

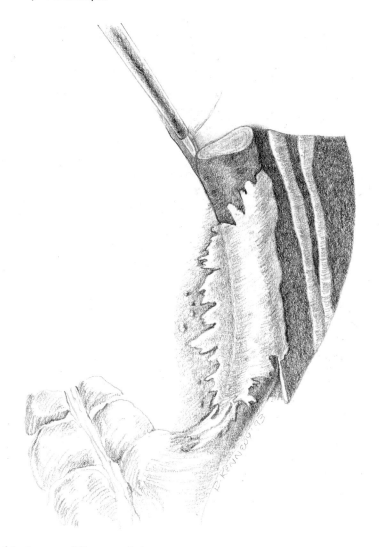

Figure 5.8 *The right uterosacral ligament is being transected at its insertion into the posterior cervix. This is carried out above all areas of fibrosis in order to ensure complete removal of invasive endometriosis in the uterosacral ligament.*

the underlying anatomy. Occasionally a vessel of the broad ligament may be lacerated. Since the peritoneum should invariably have been opened prior to such an injury, the ureter is already exposed so that coagulation of the bleeding vessel can be accomplished safely.

CONTRAINDICATIONS

If a patient is to undergo a laparoscopy, there is no known contraindication to excision other than the surgeon's inexperience. Excision can be used to treat superficial or invasive endometriosis anywhere in the body.

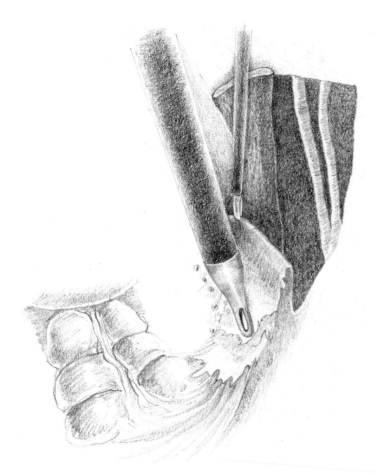

Figure 5.9 *The uterosacral ligament is shaved off the underlying pelvic floor and lateral vaginal wall attachments using 50 watts of coagulation current.*

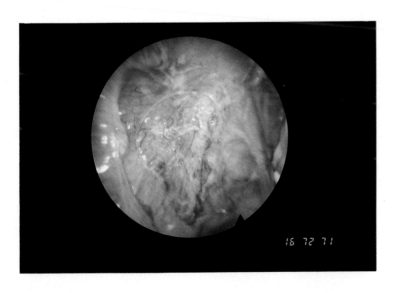

Figure 5.10 *The left uterosacral ligament has been completely resected for removal of all invasive disease.*

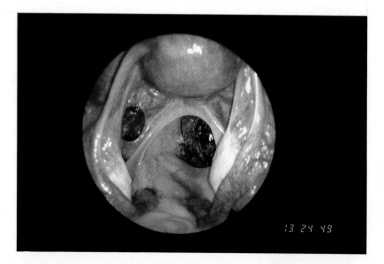

Figure 5.11 Some patients require resection of isolated areas of peritoneum for removal of superficial endometriosis.

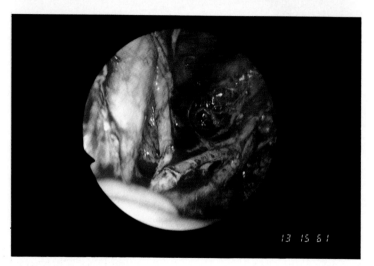

Figure 5.12 Some patients require extensive dissection of the pelvic sidewall for removal of all invasive endometriosis.

SUGGESTED READING

Redwine DB: The distribution of endometriosis in the pelvis by age groups and fertility. *Fertil Steril* 1987 **47**:173–175.

Redwine DB: Laparoscopic excision of endometriosis by sharp dissection. In Martin DC (ed) *Laparoscopic Appearance of Endometriosis*. The Resurge Press, Memphis, TN, 1990, pp. 9–19.

Redwine DB: Conservative laparoscopic excision of endometriosis by sharp dissection: life table analysis of reoperation and persistent or recurrent disease. *Fertil Steril* 1991 **56**:628–634.

Redwine DB: Treatment of endometriosis-associated pain. In Olive DL (ed) *Endometriosis: Infertility and Reproductive Medicine Clinics of North America,* WB Saunders, Philadelphia, 1992, pp. 697–720

Redwine DB: Laparoscopic excision of endometriosis by sharp dissection. In Soderstrom RA (ed) *Operative Laparoscopy, The Masters' Techniques*. Raven Press, New York, 1993, pp. 101–106.

Redwine DB: Non-laser resection of endometriosis. In Sutton CA and Diamond MP (eds) *Endoscopic Surgery for Gynaecologists*. WB Saunders, London, 1993, pp. 220–228.

6 TUBAL ECTOPIC PREGNANCY: SALPINGOSTOMY AND SALPINGECTOMY

Togas Tulandi

SALPINGOSTOMY

Early diagnosis of ectopic pregnancy has allowed conservative treatment without removing the tube. The procedure requires three or four laparoscopic punctures including a 12 mm puncture for easy removal of the specimen.

The presence of haemoperitoneum should not prevent laparoscopic treatment of ectopic pregnancy. Using a suction irrigator, the blood can be evacuated and the pelvic organs are irrigated with physiological saline or Ringer's lactate solution. Careful inspection should be done and the ectopic pregnancy is identified. The tube is immobilized with one or two laparoscopy forceps (Fig. 6.1). Using a 22-gauge injection needle inserted through a 5 mm portal, a solution of vasopressin (0.5 IU/ml of physiological saline) is injected into the mesosalpinx and into the wall of the tube at the area of maximal distention (Figs 6.2a and 6.2b). This will allow surgery with minimal bleeding. A 10–15 mm longitudinal incision is made on the maximally distended antemesosalpinx wall of the tube. This can be

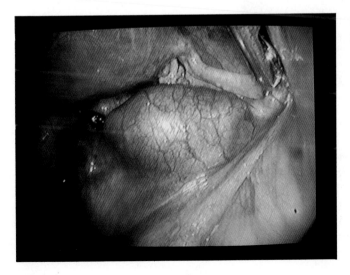

Figure 6.1 A right ampullary pregnancy.

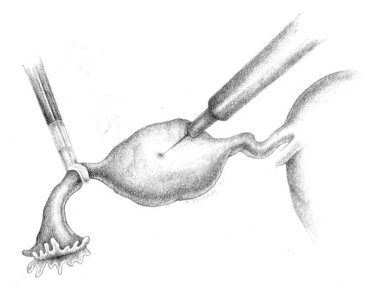

Figure 6.2a

Figures 6.2a and 6.2b *Linear salpingostomy: injection of vasopressin into the wall of the tube.*

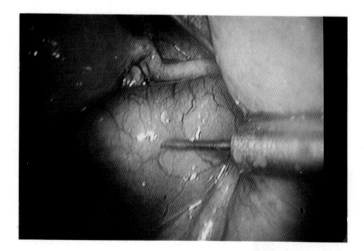

Figure 6.2b

done with either a laser with a power density of 10,000 watt/cm² for a CO_2 laser, unipolar needle electrocautery (cutting current of 10 watts) or scissors (Figs 6.3a and 6.3b). The products of conception are flushed out of the tube with a high-pressure irrigating solution. Using a combination of hydrodissection and gentle blunt dissection with a suction irrigator, the products of conception are removed from the tube (Figs 6.4a and 6.4b). This technique is preferable to piecemeal removal with forceps. The specimen is removed with 10-mm claw forceps or placed in a plastic bag (Rx Endobag, Ethicon, Inc., Somerville, NJ; Rx

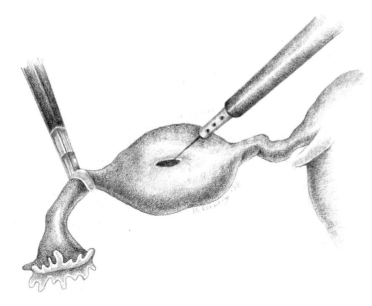

Figure 6.3a

Figures 6.3a and 6.3b *A longitudinal incision is made on the antemesosalpinx of the tube.*

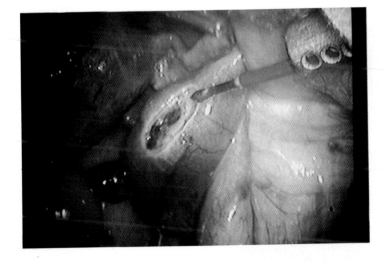

Figure 6.3b

Lapsac, Cook Ob/Gyn., Spencer, IN) and then removed from the abdominal cavity (Figs 6.5a and 6.5b).

The tube is carefully irrigated and inspected "underwater" for haemostasis. Bleeding points can be coagulated with a bipolar coagulation. The tubal incision is left open to heal by secondary intention. Before terminating the procedure, approximately 500–1000 ml of Ringer's lactate solution is left in the abdominal cavity and the pelvic organs once again inspected for accurate haemostasis ("examination underwater").

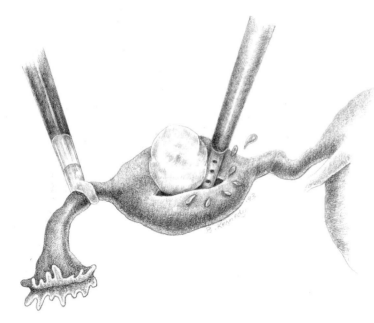

Figure 6.4a

Figures 6.4a and 6.4b *By using a suction irrigator the products of conception are flushed out of the tube.*

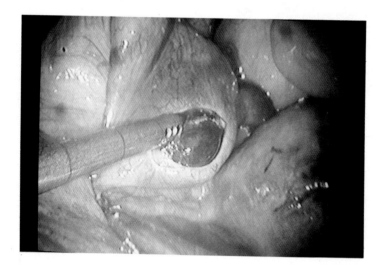

Figure 6.4b

SALPINGECTOMY

Salpingectomy with electrocautery

In the presence of persistent bleeding or rupture tubal pregnancy, a salpingectomy is an alternative. Obviously, if the patient is unstable, an immediate laparotomy should be done.

The tube is immobilized with a grasping forceps. The tubal segment to be excised is

Figure 6.5a

Figures 6.5a and 6.5b *Removal of the products of conception using claw forceps.*

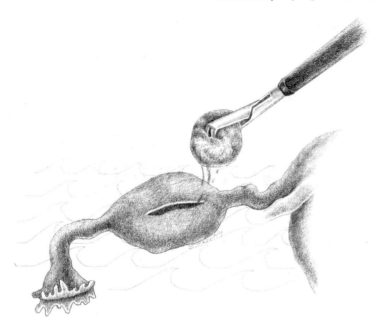

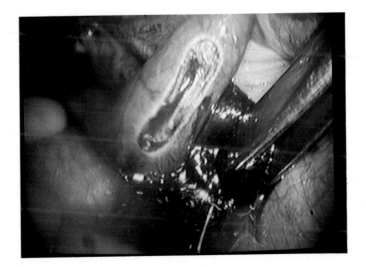

Figure 6.5b

coagulated with a bipolar cautery and cut either with laser, electrocautery or scissors (Figs 6.6 and 6.7). The procedure is repeated on the mesosalpinx of the tubal segment to be excised and on the distal portion of the tube (Figs 6.8 and 6.9). Unipolar scissors can also be used for simultaneous coagulation and cutting. Large vessels, however, have to be coagulated with bipolar forceps. Partial salpingectomy or distal salpingectomy can

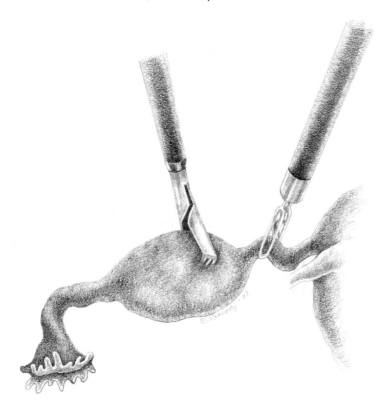

Figure 6.6 *Salpingectomy with electrocautery: coagulation of the tubal segment that will be removed.*

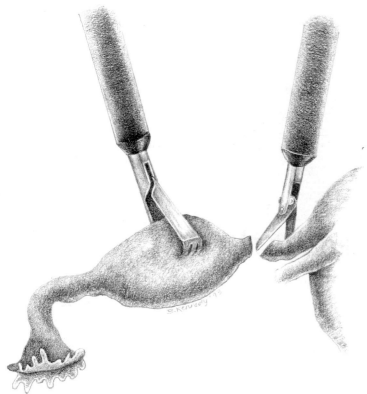

Figure 6.7 *Cutting of the coagulated tube.*

Figure 6.8

Figures 6.8 and 6.9 *The procedure is repeated on the mesosalpinx and on the distal segment of the tube.*

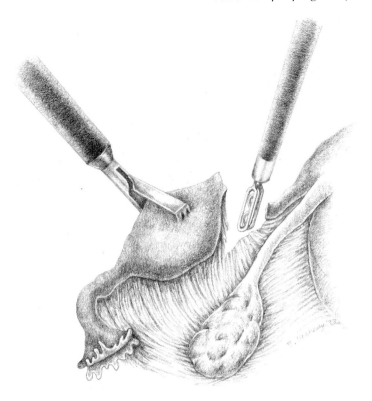

Figure 6.9

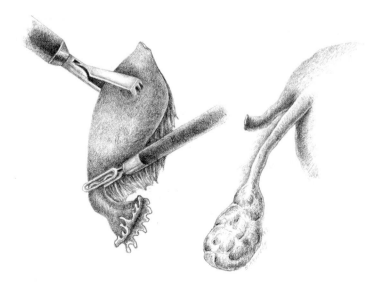

be done. The tube is removed and careful haemostasis is carried out as described above. The procedure has also been used for cornual pregnancies.

Salpingectomy with a pretied ligature (Endoloops, PercLoop)

Salpingectomy can also be achieved using a pretied ligature (Endoloops, Rx Ethicon Inc., Sommerville, NJ; PercLoop, Laparomed,

Irvine, CA). The loop is first inserted into the abdominal cavity. Grasping forceps are passed into the loop and the tube is grasped (Fig. 6.10). The portion of the tube that contains an ectopic pregnancy is lifted and a loop is placed at the base and tightened (Fig. 6.11). One or two more loops are placed above the first. The tubal segment is then cut above the loops (Fig. 6.12). If the pedicle is too large, the loop might slip. In this situation, salpingectomy with electrocautery is the preferred method.

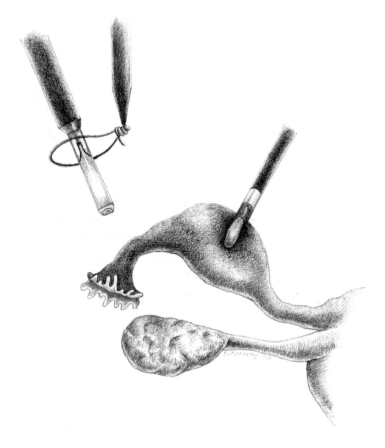

Figure 6.10 *Salpingectomy using pretied ligatures: claw forceps are passed into a pretied ligature before grasping the tubal segment to be removed.*

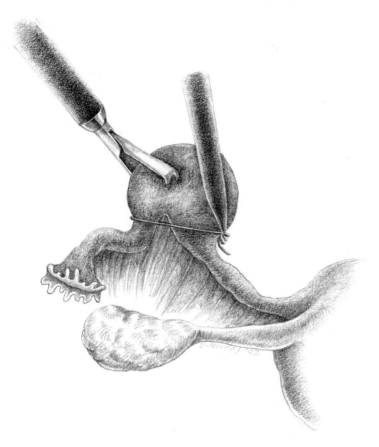

Figure 6.11 *The tube is grasped, the ligature is positioned and tightened.*

COMPLICATIONS AND THEIR PREVENTION

The possibility of leaving behind products of conception by laparoscopy is similar to that by laparotomy (up to a 5% chance). To avoid this complication, careful attention should be given to the medial portion of the tube. This is the area where the trophoblastic tissue can be inadvertently left behind causing persistent elevation of serum β-hCG levels postoperatively. In this situation, a single dose of methotrexate (1 mg/kg body weight, intramuscularly) will usually solve the problem.

CONTRAINDICATIONS

Patients who are haemodynamically unstable should undergo an immediate laparotomy.

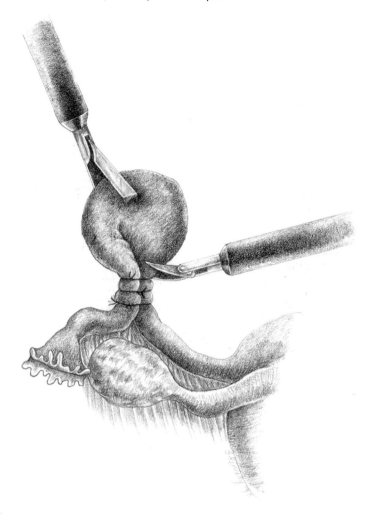

Figure 6.12 *Another one or two loops are placed above the first ligature and the tubal segment is cut above the loops.*

SUGGESTED READING

Lundorff P, Thorburn J, Lindblom B: Fertility outcome after conservative surgical treatment of ectopic pregnancy evaluated in a randomized trial. *Fertil Steril* 1992 **57:**998–1002

Pouly JL, Mahnes H, Mage G, Canis M, Bruhat MA: Conservative laparoscopic treatment of 321 ectopic pregnancies. *Fertil Steril* 1986 **46:** 1093–1097

Tulandi T: Expectant, medical or surgical treatment of tubal ectopic pregnancy. *Postgraduate Obstet Gynecol* 1992 **26:**1–6.

7 OVARIAN CYST: OVARIAN CYSTECTOMY AND PARTIAL OOPHORECTOMY

Togas Tulandi

OVARIAN CYSTECTOMY

Ovarian cysts in premenopausal age women are rarely malignant and ovarian cystectomy is a safe procedure. The incidence of malignancy is approximately 1%. It is lower in younger women and in those with a unilocular cyst. A pre-operative transvaginal ultrasound is beneficial to evaluate the type of tumour. The diagnosis is usually accurate for a functional cyst, an endometrioma or a dermoid cyst. Serum CA-125 has been used as a marker for epithelial ovarian carcinoma, but in premenopausal women it has poor sensitivity and specificity.

In the presence of an ovarian cyst the whole pelvis should be first thoroughly evaluated. Suspicious lesions should be biopsied and sent for frozen section examination. Peritoneal lavage is done and the fluid is sent for cytology. If frozen section examination is not available it is better to abandon the laparoscopy and wait for histopathological confirmation or proceed with a laparotomy. The ovarian cyst is exposed by elevating it with forceps behind the ovary or by grasping the utero-ovarian ligament (Fig. 7.1). Sometimes it is necessary for lysis of adhesions to be performed first.

The cyst is palpated with a laparoscopic probe or forceps. Using a 22-gauge injection needle inserted through a 5 mm portal, 5–10 ml physiological saline is injected into the ovarian capsule, preferably at the apex of the cyst (Figs 7.2a and 7.2b). This creates a cleavage plane by separating the capsule from the cyst wall. A superficial incision is then made on the ovarian capsule with scissors without entering the cyst (Fig. 7.3). Using a combination of hydrodissection and blunt dissection with a suction irrigator, the cleavage plane is further developed. This is usually easy to achieve especially with a dermoid cyst; but not so easy with an endometriotic cyst. Hydrodissection is done using physiological saline or Ringer's lactate solution (Figs 7.4

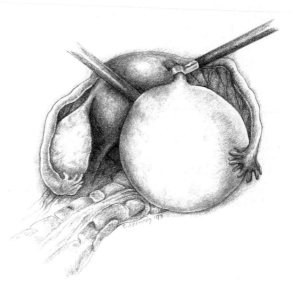

Figure 7.1 *The ovarian cyst is exposed by elevating it with forceps behind the ovary or by grasping the utero-ovarian ligament.*

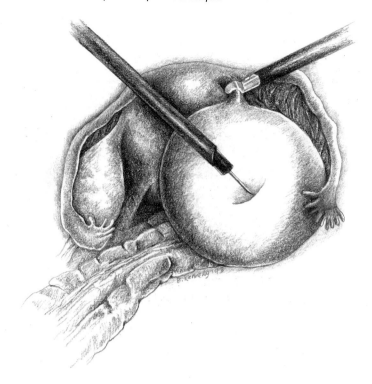

Figure 7.2a

Figures 7.2a and 7.2b *Creating a cleavage plane by injecting physiological saline into the ovarian capsule.*

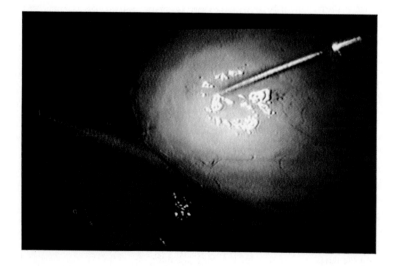

Figure 7.2b

and 7.5). The capsule is held by laparoscopic forceps and the unruptured cyst can be entirely enucleated (Figs 7.6a and 7.6b). If there is a concern of malignancy, the unruptured cyst should be inserted into a bag (Rx Endobag, Ethicon, Inc., Somerville, NJ; Lapsac, Cook Ob/Gyn., Spencer, IN), and the contents aspirated inside the bag (Fig. 7.7). The bag containing the collapsed cyst is removed via a 12 mm portal. Alternatively, it can be placed in the anterior cul de sac and aspiration with minimal spillage can be done. I usually enter the cyst with a unipolar needle electrode that is inserted into a built-in

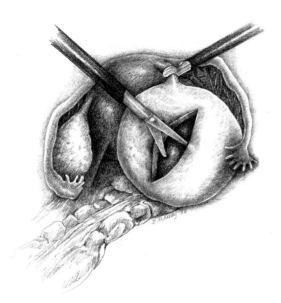

Figure 7.3 A superficial incision is made on the ovarian capsule without entering the cyst.

channel suction irrigator. The opening is then enlarged enough to fit the tip of the suction irrigator. The content of the cyst is repeatedly aspirated and diluted with the irrigating solution (Figs 7.8a and 7.8b).

Another alternative is to deliver the specimen into the vagina via a posterior colpotomy incision. Colpotomy is done by incising the vagina transversely with laser or with a unipolar needle electrode. Using a wet sponge at the end of ring forceps inside the vagina and behind the cervix, the posterior fornix is pushed upward. The incision is made transversely on the bulging vagina. The location of the rectum should be noted to avoid cutting it. Occasionally, a rectal probe is also required to ascertain that the rectum is free. The wet sponge inside the vagina prevents loss of pneumoperitoneum. If the cyst cannot be removed intact, the content of the cyst is drained through the vagina and the cyst is then removed. The colpotomy incision can be closed vaginally or laparoscopically with 2–0 polyglactin (Vicryl). Because of the possibility of contamination with vaginal flora, I rarely use this technique.

Sometimes, the cyst inadvertently ruptures during dissection. In this situation, the contents are aspirated and the cyst is repeatedly irrigated with physiological saline until clean. The inner surface of the cyst is carefully inspected for possible malignancy such as papillary projections. We found that spillage

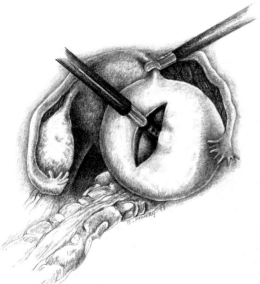

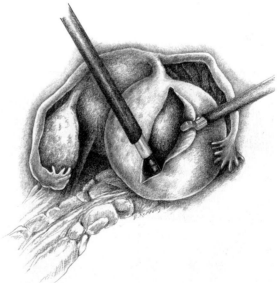

Figure 7.4

Figure 7.5

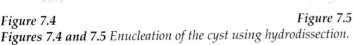

Figures 7.4 and 7.5 *Enucleation of the cyst using hydrodissection.*

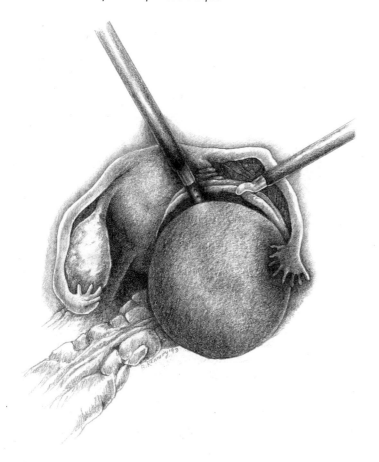

Figure 7.6a

Figures 7.6a and 7.6b *Enucleation of the cyst using hydrodissection.*

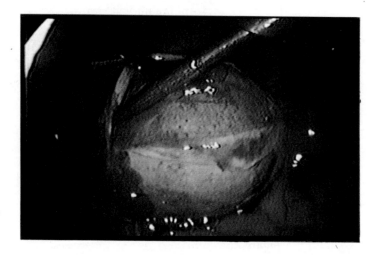

Figure 7.6b

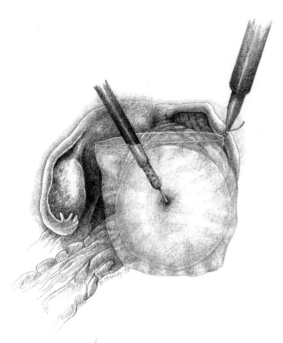

Figure 7.7 *Aspirating the contents of the cyst inside a bag.*

of the cyst's contents including that of dermoid cysts and endometrioma does not induce peritoneal reaction. This is due to liberal irrigation of the abdominal cavity. The cyst wall is then grasped with toothed forceps for traction and dissection using a combination of blunt and hydrodissection (Figs 7.9a and 7.9b). This can also be facilitated by using a "hair-curler technique". The technique is done by "curling" the cyst wall around the forceps. This movement and gentle traction will separate the cyst wall from its attachment (Fig. 7.10). Sometimes, blood vessels at the base of the cyst are found; these have to be coagulated and divided before the final removal of the cyst wall from the ovary.

The specimen is removed via a 12 mm portal (Fig. 7.11). Intermittent irrigation of the ovary allows good visualization and helps with accurate haemostasis. The ovarian defect usually collapses. However, if the ovary is gaping, two or three sutures of Vicryl 4–0 or 5–0, staples or tissue sealant can be used to approximate the edges of the ovarian tissue (Figs 7.12a and 7.12b). The ovarian capsule

can also be inverted by coagulating the inner side of the ovarian opening approximately 10 mm from its margin (Fig. 7.13). Inversion of the ovarian capsule approximates the ovarian opening.

Because ovarian cysts tend to be bilateral it is important to examine the opposite ovary. "Examination underwater" is performed at the end of the procedure to evaluate haemostasis. Approximately 500–1000 ml of Ringer's lactate solution is left in the abdominal cavity.

EXCISION (DECAPITATION) OF AN OVARIAN CYST

Occasionally, the cyst wall is so intimately adherent to the ovarian tissue that a cleavage plane cannot be created. This is not uncommonly found in ovarian endometrioma. A partial oophorectomy is an alternative. The contents of the cyst are aspirated and repeatedly irrigated. The top of the cyst, including the associated "ovarian capsule", is decapitated. Excision can be done using either a laser, unipolar scissors or a needle electrode. Care should be taken not to remove excessive ovarian tissue. After ascertaining that there are no suspicious lesions, the inner surface of the cyst wall can be destroyed either with a laser or by electrocoagulation. The ovarian tissue can be left open or closed as described above. As there is the possibility of leaving some cyst wall behind, this technique should be used rarely.

POTENTIAL COMPLICATIONS AND THEIR PREVENTION

1. The possibility of operating on an ovarian malignancy and spilling cancer cells into the peritoneal cavity can be avoided by proper selection of patients before surgery and by careful inspection at the time of laparoscopy. Peritoneal lavage and frozen section should be done for suspicious lesions.

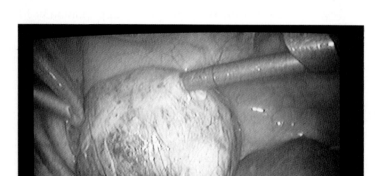

Figure 7.8a

Figures 7.8a and 7.8b *Aspiration and irrigation of an ovarian cyst at the anterior cul de sac.*

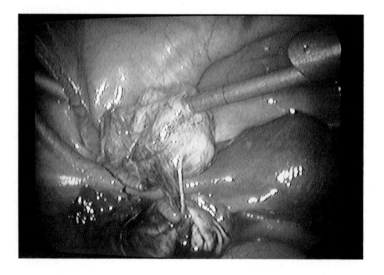

Figure 7.8b

2. Blood vessels especially at the base of the cyst should be first electrocoagulated. Although it is rarely encountered, uncontrollable bleeding requires an immediate laparotomy.

3. Potential problems due to spillage of the contents of endometrioma, mucinous cystadenoma or dermoid cyst can be eliminated by liberal irrigation of the peritoneal cavity. It is not uncommon to use 4–5 l of irrigating solution.

4. Another potential complication of ovarian cystectomy is adhesion formation. Using a meticulous technique, using non-reactive sutures (not cat-gut) and the instillation of large volumes of Ringer's lactate solution may decrease adhesion formation.

Figure 7.9a

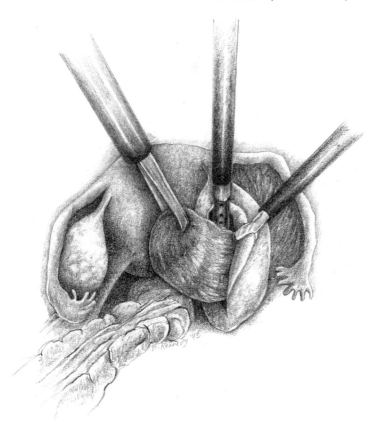

Figures 7.9a and 7.9b *A collapsed cyst wall is grasped with claw forceps for traction and dissection using blunt and hydrodissection.*

Figure 7.9b

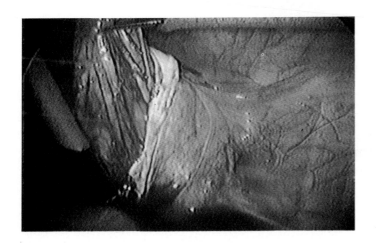

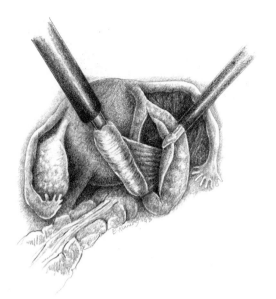

Figure 7.10 *Further separation of the cyst wall using the "hair-curler technique".*

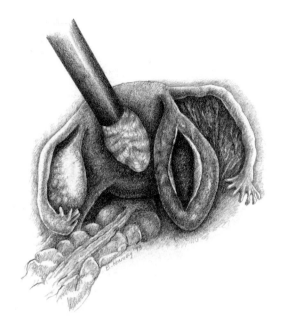

Figure 7.11 *Removal of the specimen via a 12 mm secondary portal.*

Figure 7.12a *Three sutures approximating the ovarian opening.*

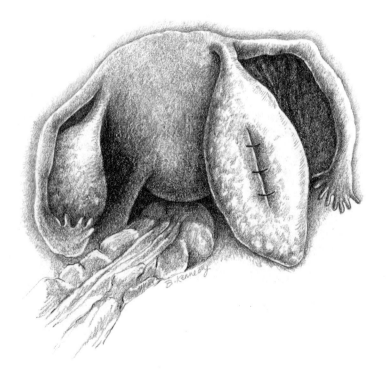

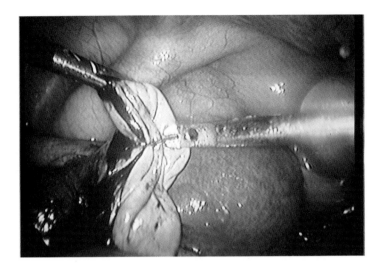

Figure 7.12b *The knot is tied using a knot pusher.*

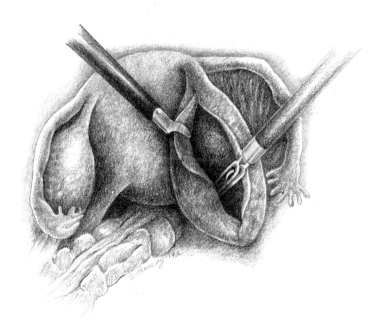

Figure 7.13 *Inversion of the ovarian opening using electrocoagulation.*

CONTRAINDICATIONS

1. Postmenopausal women with an ovarian cyst are better managed by oophorectomy.
2. Operative laparoscopy is contraindicated if there are findings of possible ovarian cancer pre-operatively or at the time of laparoscopy examination.

SUGGESTED READING

Audebert AJM: Laparoscopic ovarian surgery and ovarian torsion. In Sutton CA and Diamond MP (eds) *Endoscopic Surgery for Gynaecologists*. WB Saunders, London, 1993, pp. 134–141.

Nezhat C, Nezhat F, Welander CE, Benigno B: Four ovarian cancers diagnosed during laparoscopic management of 1,011 adnexal masses. *Am J Obstet Gynecol* 1992 **167**:790.

8 LYSIS OF ADHESIONS

Peter McComb

Preliminary assessment of the pelvis is key to successful salpingo-ovariolysis. Vital structures including intestines, blood vessels, bladder and ureter and their involvement in the distorted anatomy should be identified at the outset. Adhesions obscure structures. Proximity of the peritoneum (and vessels and ureter) to the scar tissue and differentiation between the two may be difficult.

After establishing the pneumoperitoneum, omentum may be seen to be adhered to the anterior abdominal wall and to the pelvis. It is often necessary to remove the omental adhesions before the pelvic organs can be fully visualized. Trocars are inserted at a distance and angle suitable for lysis of the omentum. The omentum tends to revascularize surrounding adherent organs and blood vessels inside the omentum tend to retract. Therefore, electrocautery and scissors are the best instruments for lysis of these adhesions.

After preliminary removal of omental adhesions, the uterus is mobilized with an intracervical cannula. The patient is placed in the Trendelenburg position and bowel is displaced towards the upper abdomen. This may be hampered by adhesions between the bowel and the pelvis. Trocars are placed about two finger breadths above the pubic symphysis. A midline and two lateral trocars are usually needed. Probes and atraumatic grasping forceps are inserted to angulate the various organs so as to assess fully the extent and type of adhesions, and to identify the organs involved. As a principle, it is better to excise the scar tissue. If the adherent structure (such as omentum) can be displaced some distance after adhesiolysis, then excision is unnecessary. If there is fusion of two organs, excision of the scar is not possible.

There are three commonly used surgical modalities: scissors, electrocautery and CO_2 laser. Unipolar electrocautery has a thermal shoulder of lateral spread of heat of greater than 2 mm, CO_2 laser has a shoulder of at least 1 mm and regular scissors have none. This allows close sharp dissection to vital and delicate structures including the tubes and ovaries. Another instrument, the suction irrigator or aquapurator (hydrodissector), can deliver Ringer's lactate solution at high pressure to the adherent tissues creating cleavage planes.

There are two basic forms of adhesions; those that are dense and fibrous, often involving a large surface area of the respective organs, and those that are filmy, flimsy and may be transparent. Lysis of these two types of adhesion from each of the pelvic organs presents unique problems.

OVARY

The ovary has a single-cell layer surface epithelium. Loss of this epithelium predisposes to scar formation. The ovary itself should not be grasped if at all possible.

Filmy adhesions

These are typically between the Fallopian tube, bowel, omentum and peritoneum or

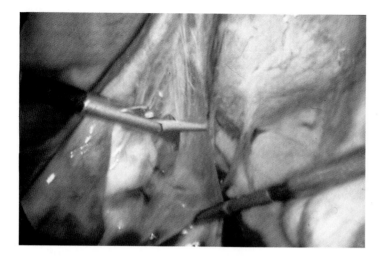

Figure 8.1 *The adhesion is stretched with a grasping forceps and then divided with scissors.*

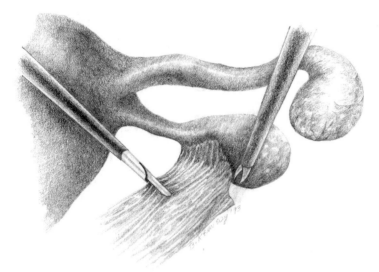

Figure 8.2 *Cutting of adhesions at the level of the ovarian surface.*

ovary. Traction is placed on the scar tissue with a grasping forceps at its attachment away from the ovary. The adhesion is angled optimally for incision (Fig. 8.1). Scissors are used to incise the adhesion at the level of the ovarian surface (Fig. 8.2). Unlike the Fallopian tube, there is no serosa to tent up from the ovary, and complete removal of the scar will facilitate ovulation. Others advocate laser or electrocautery. Any bleeding will almost always subside spontaneously. Otherwise, interstitial injection of vasopressin solution (0.5 units/ml normal saline) will assist.

Dense adhesions

Adhesions of the ovary to the pelvis, bowel to ovary, hydrosalpinx or ampulla to ovary often result in dense and fibrous adhesions. In these instances, mechanical lysis of the adhesions is the most effective procedure. Sharp incision is followed by the use of the aquapurator (hydrodissector) to establish the cleavage plane (Fig. 8.3). The aquapurator rinses the tissues free from serosanguineous fluid and assists in visualization.

If extensive raw surfaces created by the adhesiolysis are allowed to simply fall together

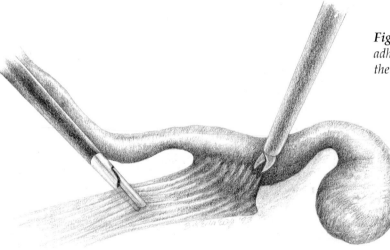

Figure 8.3 *Hydrodissection is used to establish a cleavage plane.*

Figure 8.4 *Cutting peritubal adhesions. Note that the serosa of the tube is tented.*

at the conclusion of the adhesiolysis, then scar reformation is inevitable. Suturing one organ away from the other is useful. This can be done with 6–0 polypropylene suture. Flotation of the pelvic organs by leaving 500–1000 ml of Ringer's lactate solution in the pelvis also mitigates adhesion reformation.

FALLOPIAN TUBE

Filmy adhesions

Any of the pelvic organs may be attached by filmy, flimsy transparent adhesions to the Fallopian tube. These have the potential to prevent oocyte retrieval by creating a barrier between the tube and the ovary and by limiting the motion of the fimbria. Fortunately, such adhesions are readily lysed with a low risk of reformation. Any of the three surgical modalities may be used to liberate adhesions. A peculiarity of the Fallopian tube is the loose serosa that invests the myosalpinx. When traction is applied to the scar, the serosa is tented upwards (Fig. 8.4). Care is needed to avoid incision of the serosa with denudation of the oviduct. As long as the incisions are placed at a distance from the serosa, all modalities are effective. Thermal damage of

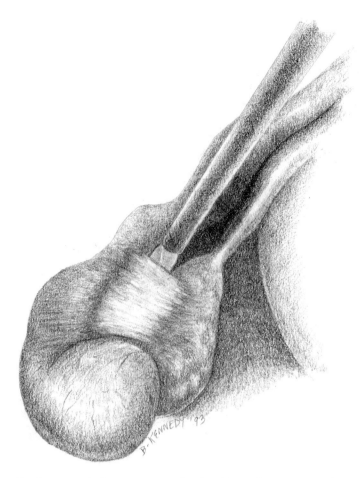

Figure 8.5 Dissection of ampullary–ovarian adhesions from the midsection of the tube towards the fimbria.

the laser and electrocautery is also limited to the scar tissue.

Dense adhesions

The tubal ampulla and hydrosalpinx are often densely adherent to the ovary. The scarring is also vascular. When the hydrosalpinx is adherent, it is necessary to distend the tube with chromopertubation dye solution to determine which part of the hydrosalpinx is fused to the ovary. It is usually the terminal portion of the tube. This tubal tissue should be carefully preserved for adequate tubal function. Ampullary–ovarian scarring is best approached by commencing the dissection from the midsection of the tube towards the fimbria (Fig. 8.5). In both instances mechanical lysis is the best. Where it is clear that there is substantial vascularity, it is prudent to have the vasopressin solution at hand.

Chromopertubation solution may leak from the hydrosalpinx into the mesosalpinx so that the mesosalpinx mimics the terminal portion of the tube. If this is not recognized, the mesosalpinx will be incised with subsequent haemorrhage. In this unenviable situation bipolar cautery and/or 6–0 polypropylene will be necessary.

POTENTIAL COMPLICATIONS AND THEIR PREVENTION

Haemorrhage is the most likely complication associated with salpingo-ovariolysis. The ability to use bipolar and unipolar electrocautery and suture at laparoscopy are key to the control of haemorrhage. The prevention of bleeding stems from an education in laparoscopic anatomy. Judicious prophylactic use of cautery, suture and vasopressor solution is also helpful in certain cases.

CONTRAINDICATIONS

1. If the surgeon feels that salpingo-ovario-lysis will not improve the patient's fertility then it should not be performed. Such cases include dense adhesions and scarring that involves extensive fusion of the peritoneal organs.
2. Proximity of the bowel, bladder and ureter to the adhesions are relative contra-indications especially in dense extensive scarring.
3. Genital tract tuberculosis is an absolute contraindication.

SUGGESTED READING

Gomel V: In Gomel V (ed) *Microsurgery in Female Infertility*. Little, Brown, Boston, PA, 1983.

McComb P: Infertility surgery: operative endo-scopy, new instruments and techniques. *Clin Obstet Gynecol* 1989 **32:**564–575.

9 ANASTOMOSIS OF THE FALLOPIAN TUBE

Peter McComb

Currently, laparoscopic tubal anastomosis should be considered experimental. However, the development of new instrumentation will allow routine conduct of tubal anastomosis by laparoscopy in the not too distant future. However, limitations will still persist. These include the thickness of the abdominal wall and the relative inability to move instruments freely through different attitudes of motion.

Surgery is performed through three 6 mm trocars placed about two finger breadths above the pubic symphysis. A midline and two lateral trocars are usually needed. The ends of the Fallopian tube are identified. There may have been a resection of a tube for an ectopic pregnancy or a previous sterilization.

The tip of each segment of occluded tube is grasped with toothed forceps and the interstitium is injected with vasopressin solution (0.5 units/ml normal saline) (Fig. 9.1). The cap of occluded tube is then excised with care to avoid the underlying vessels of the mesosalpinx (Fig. 9.2). The mesosalpinx intervening between the ends of the tubes is sewn together with 7–0 polypropylene suture. The first suture through the mesosalpinx is placed at the six o'clock position and tied (Fig. 9.3). Three additional 7–0 polypropylene sutures are then placed (Fig. 9.4). Depending on the surgeon's preference, suturing can be done extracorporeally or intracorporeally as described in Chapters 3 and 4.

In the case of an isthmic–isthmic anastomosis, the serosa is sutured with a running 7–0 polypropylene suture. In an ampullary anastomosis the sutures are placed through both the serosa and the muscularis of the tube. At the end of the procedure, the pelvis is lavaged and lactated Ringer's solution is instilled.

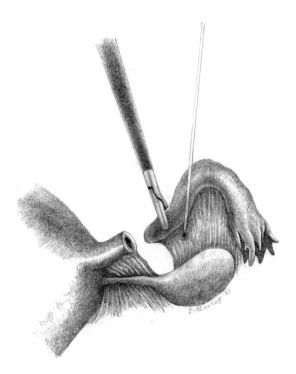

Figure 9.1 *Injection of vasopressin into the adjacent mesosalpinx.*

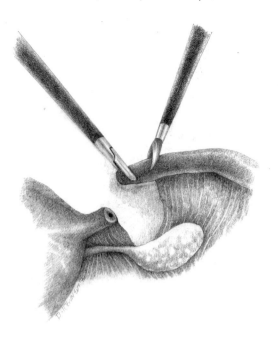

POTENTIAL COMPLICATIONS AND THEIR PREVENTION

This is a lengthy procedure, thus the surgeon must be cognizant of the risks incurred. Positioning of the patient should prevent traction of the brachial plexus and pressure on other nerves.

RELATIVE CONTRAINDICATIONS

Presently, there are no prospective randomized trials to show that anastomosis by laparoscopy is more efficacious than that by microsurgical laparotomy. To date, microsurgical tubal anastomosis by laparotomy remains the procedure of choice. Laparoscopic approach should be used only in selected cases.

Figure 9.2 Excision of the cap of occluded tube.

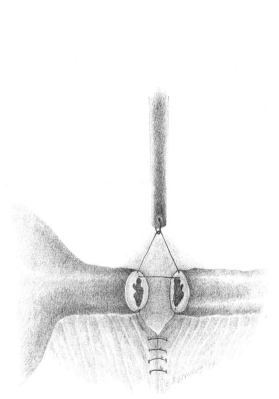

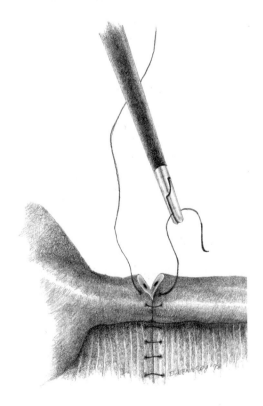

Figure 9.3   *Figure 9.4*

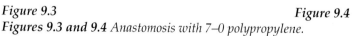

Figures 9.3 and 9.4 Anastomosis with 7–0 polypropylene.

10 SALPINGOSTOMY AND FIMBRIOPLASTY

Peter McComb

SALPINGOSTOMY

The advent of laparoscopic salpingostomy allows repair to be performed at the time of an assessment of a hydrosalpinx at laparoscopy. It is important to ascertain that there is no associated proximal tubal disease. Frequently, there are peritubal and periovarian adhesions tethering the hydrosalpinx to the ovary, and the ovary to the pelvic sidewall or other pelvic structures such as bowel and uterus. These adhesions have to be excised by scissors, electrocautery or CO_2 laser before repairing the hydrosalpinx.

Three trocars are placed suprapubically. These are 5 mm in diameter. One is on midline. The two secondary trocars are placed at the extreme limits of a generous Pfannenstiel incision.

1. Grasping forceps with a "diamond-shaped jaw" or Babcock forceps are placed on the distal ampulla of the tube, immediately adjacent to the hydrosalpinx. The hydrosalpinx is distended with transcervical chromopertubation and the pattern of scarring is observed (Fig. 10.1).

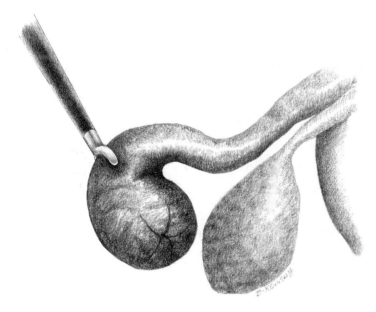

Figure 10.1 *Chromopertubation with solution of methylene blue distending the hydrosalpinx. Note the pattern of scarring.*

2. Scissors are inserted via the central trocar and the tube at the centre of the radial scars is incised. These are the sites of fusion of the fimbrial folds. Because of the associated thermal damage, I prefer not to use electrocautery or CO_2 laser (Figs 10.2a and 10.2b).

3. Scissors enter the lumen of the tube. The blades are opened to retain the scissors within the tube. The grasping forceps are transferred to the edge of the newly created ostium. The blades of the scissors are closed and the grasping forceps and scissors are spread apart to stretch and enlarge the ostium of the tube (Figs 10.3a and 10.3b).

4. Additional radial incisions open the ostium to its full extent.

5. Three or four microsutures of 6–0 polypropylene are placed around the ostium to evert the mucosal flap (Fig. 10.4). Other eversion techniques including the "Bruhat" procedure have been described. A defocused laser is applied approximately 5 mm from the margin of the mucosal flap to cause serosal contraction and

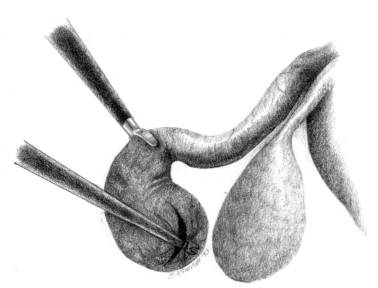

Figure 10.2a

Figures 10.2a and 10.2b Incision at the avascular line.

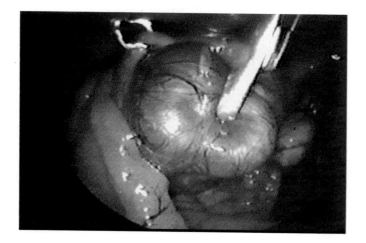

Figure 10.2b

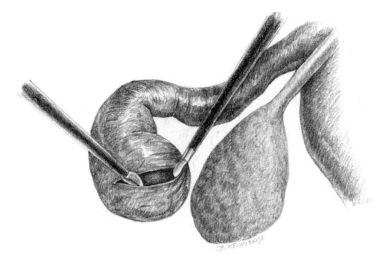

Figure 10.3a

Figures 10.3a and 10.3b
Enlargement of the neo-ostium by stretching the opening.

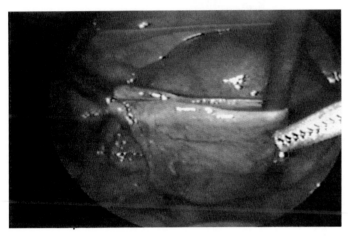

Figure 10.3b

(hopefully) eversion of the mucosal flap. Detractors of this technique point to the inevitable thermal damage to the oviduct.

6. The pelvis is lavaged and 500–1000 ml of lactated Ringer's solution is left in the peritoneal cavity.

FIMBRIOPLASTY

An identical technique is performed as for hydrosalpinx repair. It is notable that the presence of fimbrial tissue on the external surface of a phimotic tube may not be the site of the phimotic lumen (Fig. 10.5). Care is taken to locate the lumen by transcervical chromopertubation (Fig. 10.6).

POTENTIAL COMPLICATIONS AND THEIR PREVENTION

1. Haemorrhage by inadvertent incision of the mesosalpinx. This occurs when chromopertubation fluid leaks from the hydrosalpinx into the mesosalpinx. The interstitium of the mesosalpinx is distended resembling the terminus of the hydrosalpinx. If this is not recognized by the surgeon, the mesosalpinx will be inadvertently incised. The blood supply of the mesosalpinx is extensive and the vessels are relatively unsupported. Incision of these vessels can lead to profuse bleeding or haematoma formation.

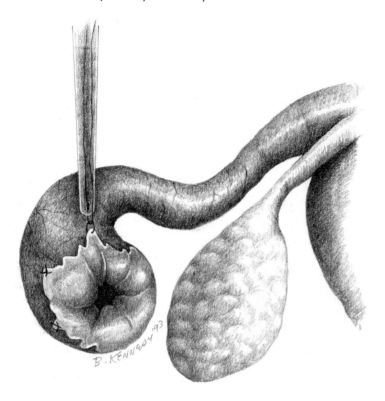

Figure 10.4 *Eversion of the mucosal flap with sutures.*

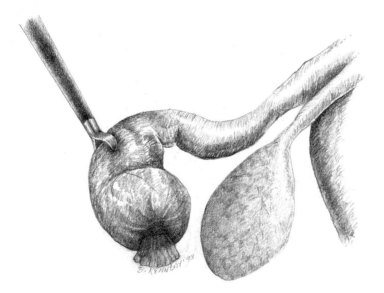

Figure 10.5 *Fimbrial tissue lateral to the phimotic ostium.*

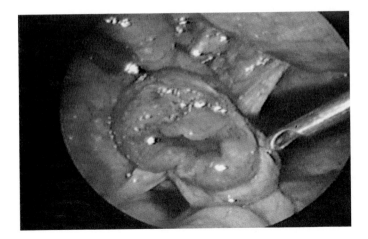

Figure 10.6 *Tubal patency is ascertained by the passage of methylene blue solution.*

2. Trauma to the tubal tissues. Excessive handling of the tube and the use of thermal energies such as laser and electrocautery may lead to scarring and tubal reocclusion. Sharp dissection is least damaging.

CONTRAINDICATIONS

If there is an associated proximal tubal disease including salpingitis isthmica nodosa and/or obstruction, further surgery is not recommended. Repair of bipolar tubal blockage (proximal and distal occlusion) rarely results in fertility.

SUGGESTED READING

Boer-Meisel ME, Te Velde ER, Habbema JDF, Kardaun JWPF: Predicting the pregnancy outcome in patients treated for hydrosalpinx: a prospective study. *Fertil Steril* 1986 **45**:23–29.

McComb P: Advances in infertility surgery: can laparoscopy replace microsurgical laparotomy? In Diamond M (ed) *Infertility Surgery*. Elsevier, New York [*Clinical Practice of Gynecology*: 1991 **3**:1–20].

11 OOPHORECTOMY AND LAPAROSCOPIC ORCHIECTOMY

Togas Tulandi

The removal of the entire ovary, especially in postmenopausal women, is sometimes indicated. Ovarian cysts in postmenopausal women or persistent pelvic pain due to ovarian endometriosis or periovarian adhesions are the possible indication for oophorectomy. Women whose first degree relatives have ovarian cancer may also benefit from bilateral oophorectomy, although this is controversial. A pre-operative transvaginal ultrasound and the measurement of serum CA-125 in postmenopausal women are indicated.

OOPHORECTOMY

In the presence of an ovarian cyst a thorough evaluation of the abdominal cavity, peritoneal cytology and a frozen section of suspicious lesions should be carried out as described in Chapter 7. Using grasping forceps, which are inserted through a secondary trocar, the ovary is grasped and pulled medially to expose the mesovarium. Using bipolar cautery, the utero-ovarian ligament is coagulated (Fig. 11.1) and then divided. While taking care to avoid the blood supply to the Fallopian tube, the same procedure is repeated on the mesovarium (Fig. 11.2) until the ovary is completely liberated. This step-by-step technique is especially valuable when the ovary cannot be freely mobilized. To increase the mobility of the ovary the broad ligament's peritoneum sometimes has to be hydrodissected away from the pelvic side wall. It is mandatory to follow the course of the ureters before commencing with a dissection. The ureters enter the pelvis by crossing the external iliac vessels close to the bifurcation of the common iliac vessels. In the pelvis, they run inferior and medial to the hypogastric vessels and then course along the lateral side of uterosacral ligaments to enter the base of the cardinal ligaments. Sometimes, the ureters have to be dissected before commencing with oophorectomy (Chapter 17).

If the ovary is not large and free, a simpler technique can be performed. The ovary is retracted medially and a pretied ligature (Endoloops, Rx Ethicon Inc., Sommerville, NJ; PercLoop, Laparomed, Irvine, CA) is placed around the mesovarium and the utero-ovarian ligament and tightened (Figs 11.3 and 11.4). One or two additional ligatures are placed above the first and the pedicle is cut with scissors. The specimen is then removed. If the specimen is too large it has to be first morcellated or cut into several pieces intra-abdominally or removed via a colpotomy incision.

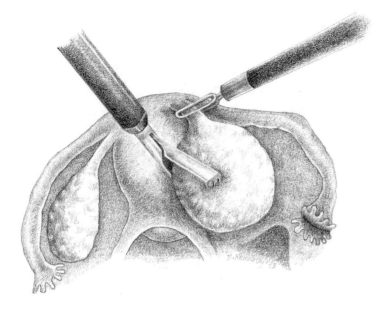

Figure 11.1 *Oophorectomy: coagulating the utero-ovarian ligament with a bipolar forceps.*

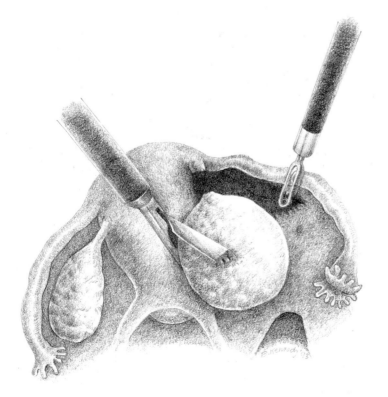

Figure 11.2 *The ovary is retracted medially with a claw forceps.*

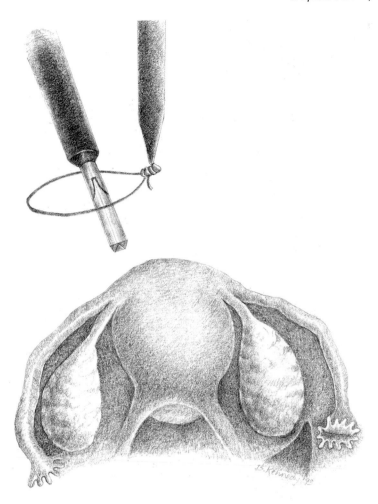

Figure 11.3 The claw forceps are passed into a pretied ligature before grasping the ovary.

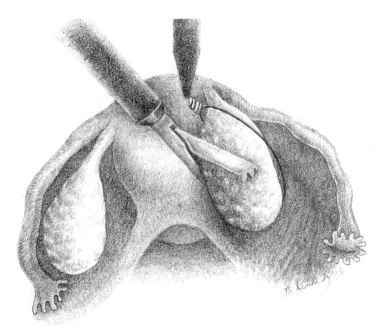

Figure 11.4 The loop around the mesovarium and the utero-ovarian ligament is tightened.

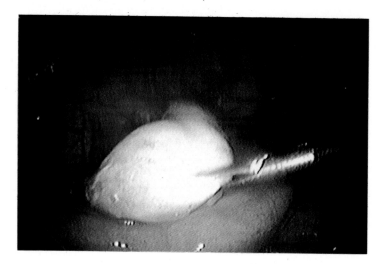

Figure 11.5 *Orchiectomy: the left testis is retracted medially with a claw forceps.*

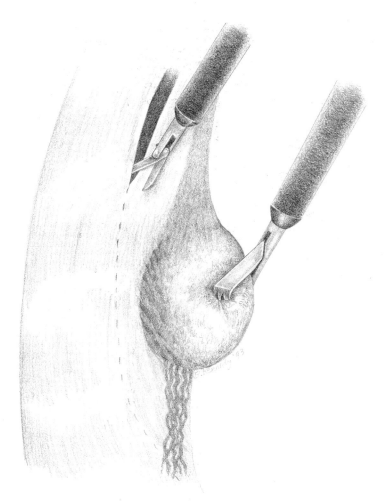

Figure 11.6 *Incision of the adjacent peritoneum lateral to the testis with unipolar scissors.*

LAPAROSCOPIC REMOVAL OF INTRA-ABDOMINAL TESTIS (ORCHIECTOMY)

Although rare, gynaecologists can encounter women with androgen insensitivity syndrome. The incidence of neoplasia in the intra-abdominal testes in these women is high (about 25%) and the gonads should be removed.

Intra-abdominal testes are usually located between the inguinal ring and the common iliac vessels. The testis is grasped with a grasping forceps and pulled medially (Figs 11.5 and 11.6). It is gradually and carefully separated from the adjacent peritoneum using unipolar scissors. The ureters are relatively far removed from the dissection area, but their course should always be followed.

The plexus pampiniformis which contains the spermatic vessels is skeletonized and two staples are placed on the vessels (Fig. 11.7). This can also be done using bipolar electrocoagulation. The pedicle is then cut between the staples. The adjacent peritoneum on the medial aspect of the testis is cut caudally until the gubernaculum is reached. Two staples are applied on the gubernaculum. It is then divided freeing the testis completely (Fig. 11.8). Pretied ligatures (Endoloops, PercLoop) can also be used. The specimen is removed.

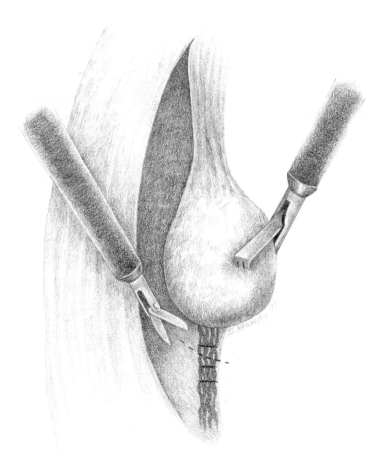

Figure 11.7 *Dividing the plexus pampiniformis between two staples. Plexus pampiniformis is located cranial to the testis.*

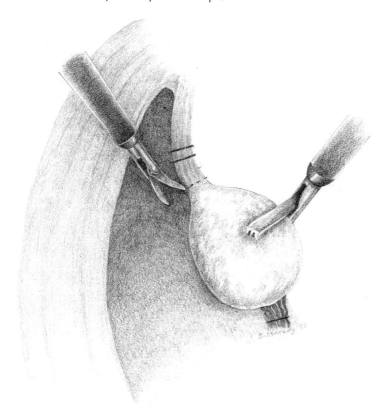

Figure 11.8 *The same procedure is done on the gubernaculum as for the plexus pampiniformis.*

COMPLICATIONS AND THEIR PREVENTION

Prevention of ureteral injury should be done by following the course of the ureter before commencing any procedure. During removal of intra-abdominal testes it is important to know the location of the iliac vessels. Potentially, these major vessels can be injured. Caudally, the bladder can be entered.

SUGGESTED READING

Bloom DA, Ayers JWT, McGuire EJ: The role of laparoscopy in the management of nonpalpable testes. *J d'Urol* 1988 **94**:465.

Daniell JF, Kurtz BR, Lee IY: Laparoscopic oophorectomy: comparative studies of ligatures, bipolar coagulation and automatic stapling devices. *Obstet Gynecol* 1992 **80**:325–328.

Kristiansen SB, Doody KJ: Laparoscopic removal of 46XY gonads located within the inguinal canals. *Fertil Steril* 1992 **58**:1076–1077.

12 LAPAROSCOPIC TREATMENT OF POLYCYSTIC OVARIAN SYNDROME

Togas Tulandi

Women with polycystic ovarian syndrome (PCOS) who are resistant to clomiphene can be treated medically with gonadotropin or surgically. The traditional surgical treatment is ovarian wedge resection. However, it requires a laparotomy and it is associated with adhesion formation. An alternative surgical treatment is laparoscopic ovarian drilling. The average ovulation rate after ovarian drilling is 80% with a conception rate of 60%.

The ovary is first immobilized by grasping the utero-ovarian ligament with grasping forceps (Fig. 12.1). Ovarian drilling can be done using continuous mode of a CO_2 laser at 25 watts or a unipolar cautery of 25–30 watts

Figure 12.1 Ovarian drilling using a unipolar needle electrode.

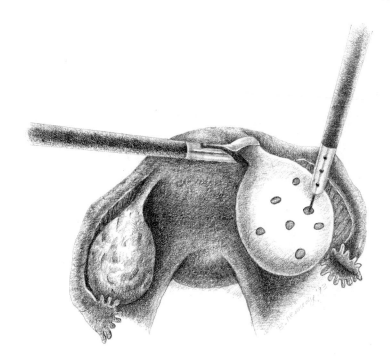

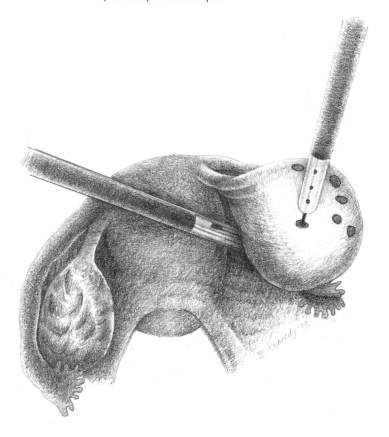

Figure 12.2 Ovarian drilling of the anterior aspect of the ovary.

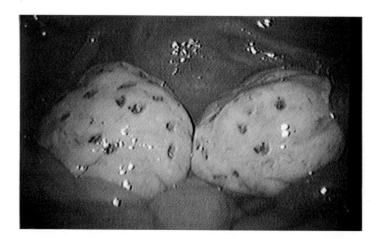

Figure 12.3 Appearance of the ovary after ovarian drilling.

with a unipolar insulated needle. As most of the uninsulated part of the needle is inside the ovary, the risk of sparking is reduced. Depending upon the size of the ovary, usually 20–30 craters in the capsule and stroma of each ovary are created. The craters are made on the subcapsular cysts. The anterior surface is exposed by "flipping" the ovary upward with forceps (Fig. 12.2). Liberal irrigation of the pelvic cavity to remove necrotic debris and carbon material should be carried out at the completion of ovarian drilling.

COMPLICATIONS AND THEIR PREVENTION

Excessive drilling may cause ovarian atrophy and premature menopause. Creating more than 30 craters per ovary and drilling the ovarian hilum should be avoided. This may jeopardize the blood supply to the ovary and may also cause bleeding. Ovarian drilling produces adhesion that may further decrease fertility. This procedure therefore should be limited to clomiphene-resistant women who for some reason cannot be treated with gonadotropin or luteinizing hormone releasing hormone.

SUGGESTED READING

Abdel Gadir A, Mowami RS, Alnaser HM *et al.*: Ovarian electrocautery, human menopausal gonadotrophins and pure follicle stimulating hormone therapy in the treatment of patients with polycystic ovarian disease. *Clin Endocrinol* 1990 **33**:585–592.

Gjonnaes H: Polycystic ovarian syndrome treated by ovarian electrocautery through the laparoscope. *Fertil Steril* 1984 **41**:20–25.

Naether OGJ, Fischer R, Weise HC, Geiger-Kötzler L, Delfs T, Rudolf K: Laparoscopic electrocoagulation of the ovarian surface in infertile patients with polycystic ovarian disease. *Fertil Steril* 1993 **60**:88–94.

13 LAPAROSCOPIC PRESACRAL NEURECTOMY

David B. Redwine

Presacral neurectomy has been performed by laparotomy since 1899. The techniques of laparoscopic presacral neurectomy have been under development since 1987. The main indication of presacral neurectomy is for attempted relief of uterine dysmenorrhoea or midline pelvic pain. Despite the term "presacral", a portion of the procedure is done on the ventral aspect of the body of the fifth lumbar vertebra as well as in the superior hollow of the sacrum.

STAGES IN THE PROCEDURE

A triple puncture technique is used, with a 10-mm operating laparoscope inserted through the umbilicus, a 5-mm grasper inserted in a left lower quadrant port lateral to the inferior epigastric vessels, and a suction irrigator inserted through a right lower quadrant port. A pair of 3-mm monopolar scissors are passed down the channel of the operating laparoscope. Laparoscopic presacral neurectomy may be done before or after any indicated pelvic surgery, although after a long case with use of copious irrigation fluid, the presacral tissue can become oedematous and the important landmarks obscured. The patient is placed in steep Trendelenburg position and the small bowel placed in the upper abdomen. The operating table is rolled to the left, displacing the sigmoid laterally. The suction irrigator is used to push the sigmoid even further laterally.

The first landmarks to identify are the major vessels in the area. While the common iliac arteries are rather obvious, the left common iliac vein and bifurcation of the vena cava extend a variable distance caudad to the aortic bifurcation (Fig. 13.1). The left common iliac vein frequently lies nearly in the midline of the promontory of the fifth lumbar vertebra, obscured by the overlying peritoneum and presacral tissue, and represents the major vascular structure which is most likely to be injured during the performance of a presacral neurectomy. The right common iliac vein lies beneath the right common iliac artery, so injury to it is less likely. The bifurcation of the vena cava and the left common iliac vein can be identified by eliciting the *waterbed sign*. Light percussion with a blunt probe of the peritoneum over the left common iliac vein will cause the low pressure blood in the vein to bounce like a waterbed.

The surgeon chooses an operative site slightly caudad to the vein. The peritoneum is grasped in the midline and elevated away from the underlying prevertebral tissue (Fig. 13.2). A touch cut is created in the peritoneum with 3-mm scissors using 70–90 watts of pure cutting current. The incision is extended transversely (Fig. 13.3) to the right common iliac vessels near the ureteral crossing, and to the base of the sigmoid mesentery on the left. Electrosurgical cutting is performed with the closed tip of the scissors, or with the edge of one blade. The scissors are not operated in a

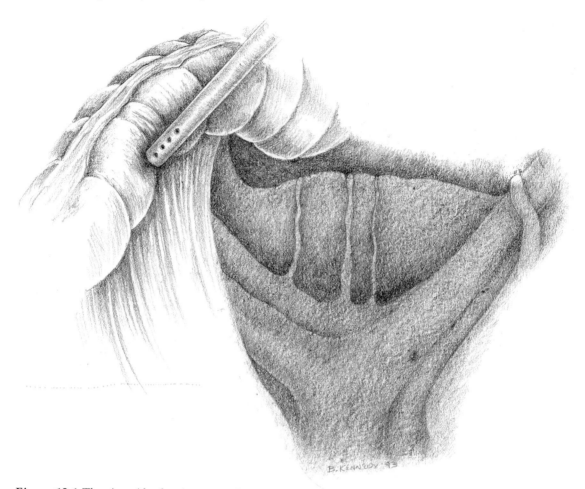

Figure 13.1 *The sigmoid colon is retracted to the left using a suction irrigator from the right lower quadrant port. The vascular structures are shown which underlie the peritoneum and the presacral tissue.*

mechanical fashion since this will result in an excessive coagulation effect rather than a clean cut.

Since the sigmoid is retracted laterally, the left margin of the dissection comes to lie in the vicinity of the left ureter. The left ureter is rarely seen during the procedure because it is hidden lateral to the vessels of the sigmoid mesentery.

After the transverse peritoneal incision is made (Fig. 13.4), blunt dissection is used at each lateral margin in order to create a window in the presacral tissue toward the periosteum. It is important to use very gentle dissection to avoid damaging the left common iliac vein. It is not necessary to blunt dissect to the periosteum in the bottom of

each window, since the purpose of creation of this retroperitoneal window is to begin to expose the underlying vascular structures for safer surgery.

Once the surgeon has confirmed the position of major retroperitoneal vascular structures by blunt dissection, a superficial layer of presacral tissue is grasped and elevated, allowing the surgeon to confirm visually that no vascular structures are elevated. The 3-mm scissors using 50 watts of coagulation current are used to transect only the elevated tissue with a touch cut, working near the rostral edge of the peritoneal incision. Working from left to right in successively deeper layers (Fig. 13.5), the presacral tissue is grasped, elevated and touch cut. By

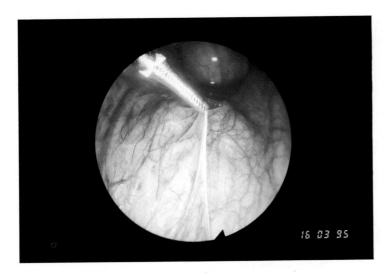

Figure 13.2 *The peritoneum is grasped and elevated away from the underlying presacral tissue. This creates a pleat of tissue in the sagittal plane which will be touch cut with 3-mm monopolar scissors. This is an entry point into the retroperitoneal space.*

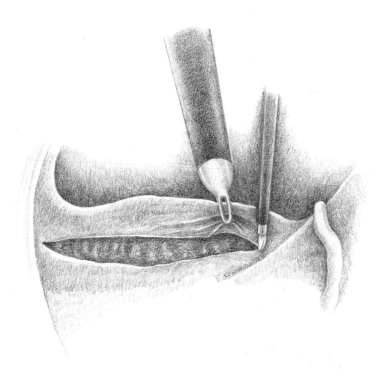

Figure 13.3 *The peritoneal incision is extended transversely from the base of the sigmoid mesentery on the left toward the right common iliac vessels and ureter on the right.*

transecting the presacral tissue in multiple small bites, damage to the underlying vascular structures can be avoided. Since it is sometimes impossible to distinguish neural tissue from fat or lymphatic tissue, it is necessary to lay the periosteum bare from the base of the sigmoid mesentery on the left (Fig. 13.5) to the right common iliac vessels and ureter on the right. Presacral veins sometimes can be found feeding into the left common iliac vein or into the bifurcation of the vena cava (Fig. 13.6). These veins can be spared with gentle dissection. Not all patients have identifiable presacral veins, and a middle sacral artery is even less commonly found.

Once the presacral tissue has been transected, its caudal cut edge can be grasped and elevated, and the presacral tissue dissected

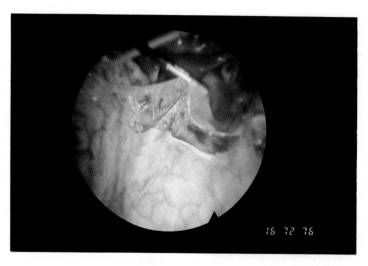

Figure 13.4 *The transverse incision through the peritoneum has been completed. It is important to avoid cutting too deep.*

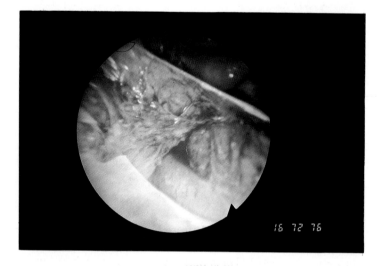

Figure 13.5 *The left margin of the dissection is shown. The left common iliac vein is seen extending caudally and to the left from the perimeter arrow in the lower right portion of the frame. Presacral veins can be seen extending across the sacral promontory and uniting with the left common iliac vein. The left common iliac vein passes beneath the mesentery of the sigmoid colon. This marks the functional left margin of the dissection. A suction irrigator can be used to push the sigmoid mesentery to the left, which will allow the left margin of the dissection to lie in the vicinity of the left ureter.*

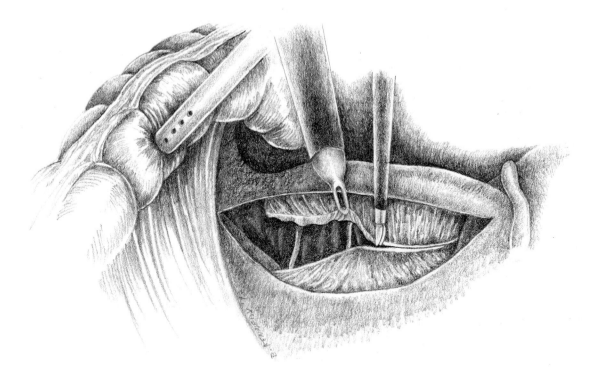

Figure 13.6 *The presacral tissue is grasped and elevated away from the underlying presacral vessels and periosteum. It is then transected in successively deeper layers from the left margin of the dissection to the right until the periosteum is bare. The presacral vessels are spared by careful dissection of the presacral tissue away from them.*

away from the periosteum and presacral vessels for several centimetres down the hollow of the sacrum. The presacral tissue is then bluntly stripped from the overlying peritoneum (Fig. 13.7) and transected distally using 50 watts of coagulation current (Fig. 13.8). At this point, care must be taken not to coagulate blindly through the overlying peritoneum since the sigmoid colon is always present immediately behind the peritoneum. At the conclusion of the procedure, the periosteum has been laid completely bare from the base of the sigmoid mesentery to the right common iliac vessels. Retroperitoneal tissue has been stripped from the right common iliac vessels to the right ureter (Fig. 13.9).

POTENTIAL COMPLICATIONS

Damage to the left common iliac vein or presacral veins will likely occur if the presacral tissue is transected with imprecise energy sources such as the argon beam coagulator or CO_2 laser. If these energy sources are used, a backstop is recommended to protect the major vessels. If inadequate retroperitoneal dissection is performed, or if large bundles of presacral tissue are grasped greedily, damage to surrounding structures is more likely to occur. Vigorous dissection in the sigmoid mesentery can result in significant bleeding, and subsequent coagulation to control bleeding could damage the hidden left ureter.

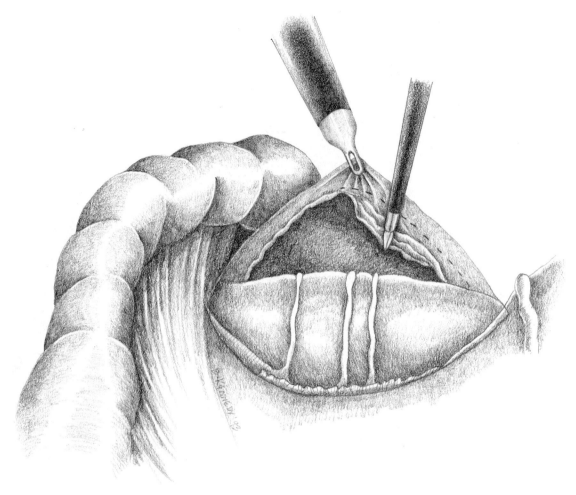

Figure 13.7 *The presacral tissue is now stripped from the overlying peritoneum using blunt dissection.*

Post-operatively, patients may rarely have a decreased sense of bladder fullness, although this could be a uterine effect rather than a bladder effect. Urgency is rarely seen. The majority of patients have no change in bowel or bladder function.

CONTRAINDICATIONS

Although there are no specific contra-indications, obese patients have more retroperitoneal fatty tissue in the presacral area. This can increase the difficulty of surgery and rarely may cause abandonment of the procedure.

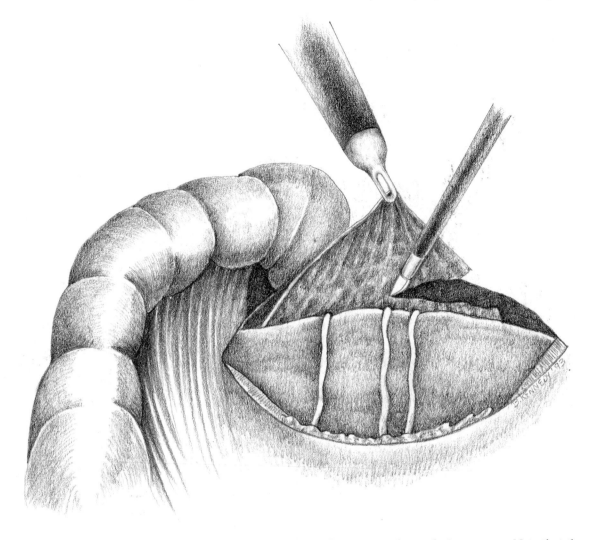

Figure 13.8 *The presacral tissue is transected distally with 50 watts of coagulating current. Note that the sigmoid colon lies just beyond the peritoneum.*

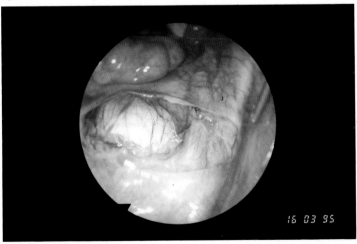

Figure 13.9 *The right margin of the dissection is shown at the conclusion of the procedure. The right common iliac vein and artery are seen. The right ureter crosses the right common iliac artery at the right angle of the peritoneal incision.*

SUGGESTED READING

Candiani G, Fedele L, Vercellini P, Bianchi S, DiNola G: Presacral neurectomy for the treatment of pelvic pain associated with endometriosis: a controlled study. *Obstet Gynecol* 1992 **167**:100–103.

Jaboulay M: Le traitement de la neuralgie pelvienne par la paralysie du sympathique sacre. *Lyon Med* 1899 **90**:102–108.

Lee RB, Sonte K, Magelssen D, Belts RP, Benson WL: Presacral neurectomy for chronic pelvic pain. *Obstet Gynecol* 1986 **68**:517–521.

Nezhat C, Nezhat F: A simplified method of laparoscopic presacral neurectomy for treatment of central pelvic pain due to endometriosis. *Br J Obstet Gynaecol* 1992 **99**:659–663.

Perez JJ: Laparoscopic presacral neurectomy. Results of the first 25 cases. *J Reprod Med* 1990 **35**:625–630.

Polan ML, DeCherney A: Presacral neurectomy for pelvic pain in infertility. *Fertil Steril* 1980 **34**:557–560.

Redwine DB: Laparoscopic presacral neurectomy (video). In *The Video Journal of Obstetrics and Gynecology*. Medical Video Productions, St Louis, May, 1991.

Redwine DB, Perez JJ: Laparoscopic presacral neurectomy. In Soderstrom RA (ed) *Operative Laparoscopy, The Masters' Techniques*. Raven Press, New York, 1993 pp. 157–160.

Tjaden B, Schlaff WD, Kimball, Rock JA: The efficacy of presacral neurectomy for the relief of midline dysmenorrhea. *Obstet Gynecol* 1990 **76**:89–91.

14 LAPAROSCOPIC UTERINE NERVE ABLATION (LUNA)

Togas Tulandi

The sensory nerve fibres from the uterus and cervix traverse the Frankenhauser plexus which is located in, under and around the uterosacral ligament's attachment to the posterior wall of the cervix. Ablation of the uterosacral ligaments will disrupt the continuity of these nerve fibres. Pain relief has been reported in about 70% of patients treated by LUNA.

The ureter is located close to the uterosacral ligament and because of this the posterior broad ligaments should be carefully inspected to identify the course of the ureters. They are usually located 10–20 mm lateral to the uterosacral ligaments. Peristaltic movements of the ureters can be elicited by palpating the ureters with an atraumatic forceps. The uterosacral ligaments are exposed by elevating the uterus with a uterine manipulator. Sometimes, the ligaments are attenuated and not clearly defined. In this situation, either a suction irrigator or laparoscopic forceps are pushed against the posterior aspect of the cervix to tent up the ligaments (Fig. 14.1).

The course of the ureters is inspected again

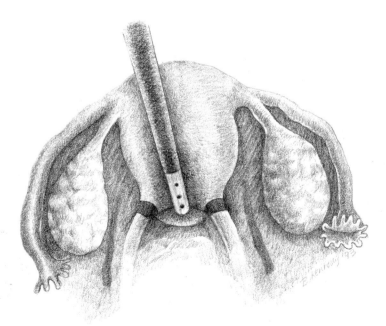

Figure 14.1 Exposing the uterosacral ligaments with a suction irrigator during the ablation. Note the course of the ureters (dark shadow) lateral to the ligaments.

and ablation of the uterosacral ligaments is done using laser (power density 10,000 watts/cm^2) or unipolar cautery scissors. Bipolar coagulation and sharp dissection can also be done. Ablation is carried out perpendicular to the ligaments as close to the cervix as possible at their attachment to the cervix. A crater 5 mm deep and 10 mm in diameter is created. Attention should be given not to injure the ureters, blood vessels on the lateral aspect of the ligaments and the rectum. Interruption of crossing nerve fibres between the two ligaments can be done by lasering or electrocoagulating the area between the two craters superficially. At the completion of the procedure the pelvic cavity should be irrigated. The irrigation removes any necrotic debris and carbon material produced. "Examination underwater" is performed to ascertain that there is no bleeding.

POTENTIAL COMPLICATIONS AND THEIR PREVENTION

LUNA is a simple procedure. However, it can lead to a catastrophic complication of transecting the ureters, rectal injury, major bleeding and even death. Ureteral injury should be immediately recognized and repaired. It is of paramount importance to identify the ureters and blood vessels lateral to the uterosacral ligaments before performing LUNA. Bleeding can also occur because the transection is made too deep. This can usually be controlled by bipolar electrocoagulation.

SUGGESTED READING

Daniell JF: Fiberoptic laser laparoscopy. In Sutton C (ed) *Baillière's Clinical Obstetrics and Gynaecology. Laparoscopic Surgery* 1993 **3(3):** 545–562.

15 MYOMECTOMY

Peter McComb

Myomectomy is an operation that can be performed by laparoscopy. However, there are circumstances when this operation is not indicated. These circumstances include:

1. Multiple fibroids that may preclude detection and removal at laparoscopy.
2. Fibroids greater than 100 mm in diameter. The removal of such tumours is time consuming.
3. Suspicion of malignancy. This includes the situation when a "fibroid" treated by gonadotropin releasing hormone analogue has led to vaginal bleeding.
4. Fibroids in locations that are inaccessible to the laparoscope. These may include deep intramural or submucosal or intracavitary fibroids, cervical fibroids and broad ligament fibroids.
5. Instances when a laparotomy is otherwise indicated for associated diseases, for example, ovarian neoplasia.

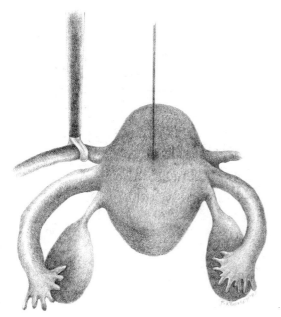

Figure 15.1 *Injection of vasopressin into the pseudocapsule of the myoma.*

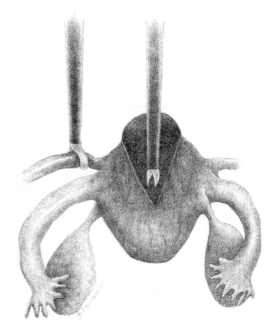

Figure 15.2 *Incision of the myometrium.*

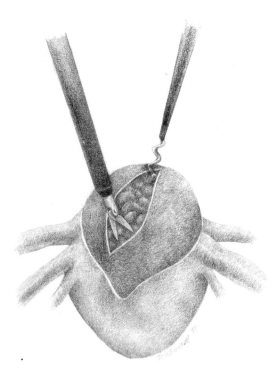

Figure 15.3 *Myoma enucleation with the help of a myoma screw.*

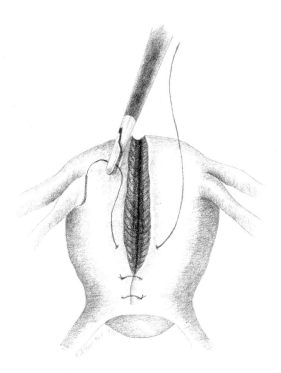

Figure 15.5 *Repair of myoma incision.*

Pre-operative hysterosalpingography and transvaginal ultrasonography are the minimal prerequisite pre-operative investigations. Two trocars of 5 mm and one of 12 mm for tissue removal are required.

1. The uterus is stabilized with "diamond-jaw" grasping forceps applied to the round ligament or ovarian ligament. A solution of vasopressin (0.5 units/ml of physiological saline) is then injected into the myometrium adjacent to the myoma via a transabdominal 22-gauge spinal needle or a laparoscopic injection needle. Up to 10 ml of this solution may be injected during the procedure (Fig. 15.1).
2. The myometrium directly over the fibroid is incised with hook scissors (Fig. 15.2).
3. The incision is deepened into the substance of the fibroid to permit toothed grasping forceps to gain purchase and grasp the fibroid tissues. Alternatively, a "myoma screw", a corkscrew mounted on a rod, may be spiralled into the fibroid to provide traction (Fig. 15.3).

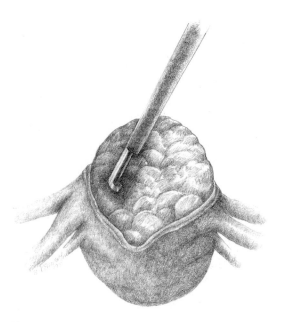

Figure 15.4 *Morcellation of an intramural myoma with a morcellator.*

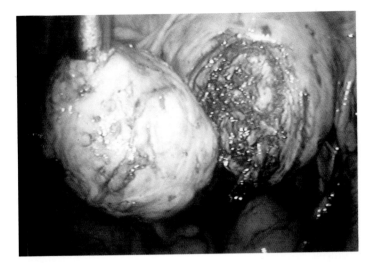

Figure 15.6 An intramural myoma has been enucleated (courtesy of Dr H. C. Topel).

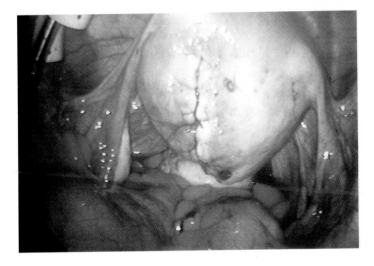

Figure 15.7 The uterine defect has been sutured (courtesy of Dr H. C. Topel).

4. Traction is placed on the fibroid to withdraw it from the uterus. Scissors and blunt dissecting forceps separate the fibroid from the surrounding myometrium.
5. If a morcellator is to be used, the fibroid is left partially attached to the uterus to stabilize the tissue during morcellation (Fig. 15.4).
6. The uterine incision is repaired with 2–0 polypropylene for the myometrial repair, and 6–0 polypropylene for the closure of the uterine serosa (Fig. 15.5). A knot pusher is used to apply extracorporeal knots to the tissues.
7. The specimen can be removed via a posterior colpotomy opening. The fibroid is applied to the colpotomy opening, grasped with a transvaginal tenaculum and withdrawn from the peritoneal cavity.

POTENTIAL COMPLICATIONS AND THEIR PREVENTION

1. Haemorrhage may complicate a laparoscopic myomectomy. For this reason, only fibroids that are fully accessible to the peritoneal cavity should be approached laparoscopically. Removal of myomata that are deep in the myometrium or within the broad ligament may be complicated by bleeding that is difficult to control.

2. Adhesions frequently complicate myomectomy. The laparoscopic environment is
conducive to excellent wound healing.
Nevertheless, it is important to close the
serosal layer with fine non-reactive suture
(6–0 or lighter) to avoid adhesion
formation.

3. Uterine rupture in pregnancy and uterine
decapitation a few weeks following a
laparoscopic myomectomy have been
reported. Proper closure of the uterine wall
is therefore mandatory.

CONTRAINDICATIONS

Contraindications include multiple fibroids,
large fibroids (greater than 100 mm), suspected
malignancy, inaccessible fibroids and
instances when a laparotomy is otherwise
indicated.

SUGGESTED READING

Hasson HM, Rotman C, Rana N, Sistos F,
Dmowski WP: Laparoscopic myomectomy.
Obstet Gynecol 1992 **80**:884–888.

Tulandi T: The role of laparoscopy in the management of leiomyomata uteri. *SOGC Journal* (in
press).

Verkauf BS: Myomectomy for fertility enhance-
ment and preservation. *Fertil Steril* 1992 **58**:1–15.

16 LAPAROSCOPIC PELVIC AND AORTIC LYMPHADENECTOMY

Nicholas Kadar and Harry Reich

Pelvic and/or aortic lymphadenectomy are central to the surgical management of many patients with gynaecological malignancies. Both procedures can be performed laparoscopically and the morbidity is lower than after an open operation. The question to be directed at laparoscopic lymphadenectomy is simply whether it can achieve what can be accomplished with the open operation. The indications for laparoscopic lymphadenectomy should be exactly the same as they are for the open operation, and differences of opinion concerning these indications is no argument against the use of the laparoscopic route.

ADEQUACY OF LAPAROSCOPIC LYMPHADENECTOMY

The adequacy of laparoscopic lymphadenectomy *vis-à-vis* the open operation must be determined by comparing the number of lymph nodes removed and the proportion of patients found to have nodal disease after each type of procedure. The same type of dissection should be done either by laparoscopy or by laparotomy. The completeness of the procedure can be evaluated by taking photographs at the completion of the dissection.

PELVIC LYMPHADENECTOMY

Kadar appears to have been the first to perform a complete pelvic lymphadenectomy laparoscopically for gynaecological malignancies, a procedure that requires mobilization of the iliac vessels from the psoas muscle (Fig. 16.1), separation of the iliac artery and vein, and their "skeletonization" (Fig. 16.2). The average number of nodes recovered by the author from patients with stage IA2-IIA carcinoma of the cervix treated by laparoscopically assisted radical vaginal hysterectomy and pelvic lymphadenectomy was 30.9. Although Childers and colleagues have performed the largest number of laparoscopic lymphadenectomies, they did not attempt complete lymphadenectomies laparoscopically until they had performed almost 100 cases.

AORTIC LYMPHADENECTOMY

In our series of patients undergoing laparoscopic aortic lymphadenectomy for advanced cervix cancer the average number of nodes recovered was 12.8, and 60% of patients have had positive nodes; figures that clearly equal those reported for the open operation. We have also been able laparoscopically to resect nodes that were fixed to great vessels, and extend the dissection to the renal vein if necessary. Unlike others, we have not found the left-sided dissection to be any more difficult

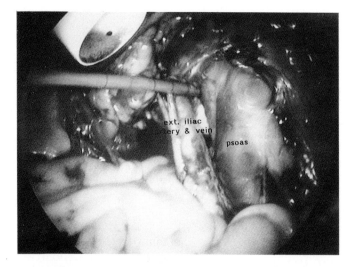

Figure 16.1 *Laparoscopic pelvic lymphadenectomy. Nodal tissue has been removed from in front of the psoas muscle and external iliac artery, and the external iliac vessels are being mobilized from the psoas muscle.*

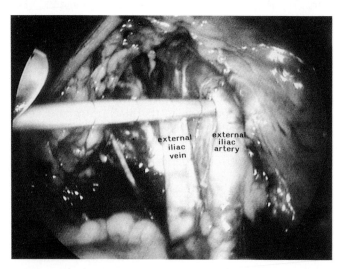

Figure 16.2 *The areolar sheaths around the external iliac vessels have been removed and the vessels separated.*

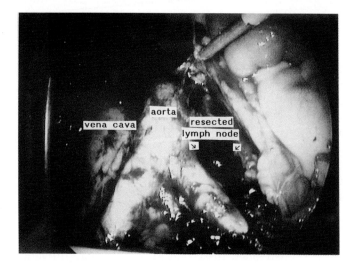

Figure 16.3 *Bilateral, laparoscopic inframesenteric aortic lymphadenectomy in a patient with stage IIIB cancer of the cervix. The "bed" of a large 50 mm lymph node containing metastatic disease can be seen to the left of the lower aorta.*

or problematic than the right side and in fact one patient had a fixed, 50-mm lymph node resected from the left side of the aorta (Fig. 16.3).

OPERATIVE TECHNIQUES

Preliminaries

Patients are positioned awake in the Allen stirrups with the knees flexed, and the thighs abducted, but not flexed at the hips, for all laparoscopic operations. However, for laparoscopic aortic lymphadenectomy, they are placed flat on the operating table. One of us (NK) prefers to pass ureteric stents routinely because they make the ureters much more prominent and aid in their identification and retraction. (The purpose of the stent is *not* to help "palpate" the ureter endoscopically with instruments.)

The following trocar placements are used (Fig. 16.4): the laparoscope is passed through a 10 mm umbilical or sub-umbilical port, a 10 mm port is placed supra-pubically, and a 5 mm port is placed on either side of the rectus muscles just above a line joining the anterior superior iliac spines. For aortic lymphadenectomy, an additional 5 mm port is needed for retraction, and it is placed just below the ribs (and liver) to the right of the falciform ligament.

Sharp scissor dissection and a two-handed approach is used throughout. The right-handed surgeon holds a grasper in the left hand, and uses it as a dissecting forceps, and the assistant holds the camera. Bleeding is controlled mostly with an unblended monopolar current, but larger perforating vessels to the vena cava or aorta, or an aberrant obturator vein, need to be clipped or desiccated with a bipolar current. If the ovarian artery or vein needs to be divided they are clipped prior to division.

Figure 16.4 Trocar placement used for laparoscopic radical pelvic surgery.

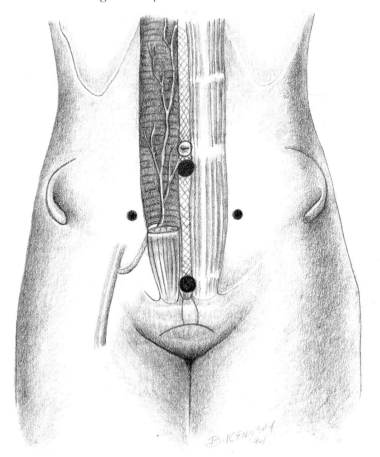

Laparoscopic pelvic lymphadenectomy

Laparoscopic pelvic lymphadenectomy can proceed in exactly the same way as the open operation. Indeed, the surgeon will find that he or she obtains a far better view of the obturator fossa than at laparotomy. The pelvic spaces are first developed and ureters identified as described in Chapter 17. The surgical limits of the dissection are then delineated. These are: the *common iliac artery* proximally (i.e. cephalad), the *psoas muscle* laterally, the *circumflex iliac vein* and pubic bone distally (i.e. caudad) the *obliterated umbilical artery* medially, and the *obturator fossa* inferiorly (i.e. ventrally). There are five steps in the operation:

Step 1. Separating the external iliac vessels from the psoas muscle and entering the obturator fossa lateral to the vessels

To mobilize the external iliac vessels, the dense areolar tissue that attaches the vessels to the psoas muscle is scored very superficially with scissors from the common iliac artery all the way down to the circumflex iliac vein. The incision must be very superficial to avoid injury to the vein which lies just below the artery. Using blunt dissection with the back of the dissecting scissors or dissecting forceps, the external iliac artery and vein are peeled off the psoas muscle. Once the vein is freed, with progressively deeper dissection the surgeon will gain entry into the obturator fossa, identified by the bright yellow fatty-nodal tissue that comes into view. By continuing the plane of dissection lateral to this tissue, the nodal tissue in the obturator fossa is mobilized medially. There are no branches lateral to the external iliac artery or vein, but very occasionally nutrient muscular branches can be encountered which can be safely coagulated or clipped.

Step 2. Freeing the external iliac artery and vein from the areolar sheath and separating the vessels

The external iliac artery and vein are next freed from their areolar investments. Each vessel is completely surrounded by its own distinct areolar sheath, and the two sheaths are fused along the entire course of the vessels. The sheath of the external iliac artery is incised with scissors along its dorsal surface from the level of the common iliac artery all the way down to the circumflex iliac vein. There are no branches of the artery in this region but some hair-like vessels in the arterial sheath may need to be coagulated. The medial border of the sheath is grasped with dissecting forceps and the artery is freed from its areolar investment mostly with blunt dissection but cutting areolar attachments as needed.

At this point, the sheaths of the external iliac artery and vein are still joined along the undersurface of the artery, and the next step is cautiously to incise the sheath of the external iliac vein. It is this step which requires the greatest care in the entire dissection, as the edge of the vessel can easily be compressed and merge imperceptibly with the areolar sheath that covers it. However, once a nick has been made in the sheath, the glistening surface of the vein becomes unmistakably clear and distinct from its areolar covering. The same technique of sharp and blunt dissection can then be used to free the vein circumferentially from its sheath. The final step in this part of the dissection is to free the inferior border of the vein which is tethered by loose areolar tissue to the pelvic side wall and obturator fossa. This is done mainly to gain free access to the obturator fossa. Occasionally, an aberrant obturator vein is encountered coursing upwards to enter the external iliac vein. It has to be clipped and divided.

Step 3. Removal of fatty-node-bearing tissue from the front of the psoas muscle and the external iliac vessels

The fatty-nodal tissue in front of the psoas muscle and external iliac vessels is next removed by grasping the tissue with spoon forceps and freeing its areolar attachments with sharp scissor dissection. If this tissue is abundant and obscures view of the iliac vessels and psoas, it may need to be removed at the start of the lymphadenectomy. The nodes in this region are distributed along the course of the external iliac artery in a cephalad–caudad direction, and are attached laterally to the psoas muscle and medially to the sheath of the external iliac artery by loose areolar tissue. Distally, at the level of the circumflex iliac vein, there are quite prominent nodes lying in a lateral–medial direction across the lower part of the external iliac artery. The most lateral part of this nodal bundle is about 20–30 mm from the artery, and has a nutrient branch which has to be coagulated first. The medial attachments of these nodes are freed when the external iliac vessels are dissected from their sheaths; all that remains then, is to free their lateral attachments to the psoas muscle. As this is done, the ilio-femoral and genito-femoral nerves are encountered and they can easily be pushed laterally.

Step 4. Freeing the obturator nerve from the fatty-nodal bundle in the obturator fossa and dissection of the obturator nodes from the pubic bone, the internal iliac artery until the bifurcation of the iliac artery

Finally, the obturator fossa and internal iliac vessels are freed. This is best done by retracting the external iliac vessels laterally, and teasing out the obturator nerve from the most inferior part of the obturator nodal bundle using the closed tips of the dissecting scissors. Once the nerve is freed, the distal attachments of the nodal bundle can be freed from the pubic bone by dividing them with a cutting current. The nodal bundle is then grasped with spoon forceps, elevated and placed on tension. It is then teased off its most ventral attachments below the obturator nerve using a gentle sweeping motion with the partly opened scissors. As this nodal tissue is freed in a cephalad direction, residual attachments to the external iliac vein usually need to be freed. Ultimately, the internal iliac artery is reached, and the nodal tissue lying anteriorly, laterally and medially is freed in continuity with the obturator fossa nodal mass. The nodal tissue can be quite adherent in this region because the internal iliac artery does not have an areolar sheath as do the external iliac vessels.

Step 5. Retraction of the external iliac vein laterally to ensure that the bifurcation of the iliac artery has been completely cleared of node-bearing tissue

With further dissection in a cephalad direction, the bifurcation of the iliac artery is reached, and this region must be cleaned with care. Note that the external and internal iliac veins lie just laterally. Any nodal tissue lying lateral to and in front of the lower part of the common iliac artery is also usually freed at this point, although it can also be removed at the start of the lymphadenectomy. Once the attachments of the nodal bundle in this region are divided, the dissection is complete (Fig. 16.5).

Laparoscopic aortic lymphadenectomy

After pneumoperitoneum and insertion of the trocars, the patient is positioned in the steep Trendelenburg position and rotated slightly to her left. The abdomen and pelvis are inspected, peritoneal washings are taken, the sigmoid colon is retracted laterally, small bowel is displaced from the pelvis, and the root of the mesentery is elevated. The posterior parietal peritoneum is opened in one of several ways: over the right common iliac artery, medial to the right ureter; parallel to the small bowel mesentery; vertically downwards in the midline from the root of the mesentery, or in the reverse direction, starting above the sacral promontory, medial to the sigmoid mesentery. The peritoneum is incised with scissors, and using mostly blunt dissection, a plane is developed between the peritoneum and the node-bearing fatty areolar tissue overlying the great vessels. It is important to develop this plane properly and widely before carrying the dissection down to the adventitia of the aorta. Otherwise the nodal tissue may be elevated with the bowel mesentery and the retroperitoneal fat during retraction, and the nodes will not be removed.

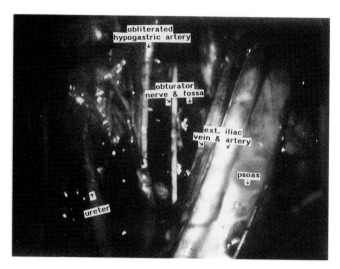

Figure 16.5 Completed laparoscopic pelvic lymphadenectomy.

The node-bearing areolar tissue in front of the aorta is then incised and the incision is carried down to the adventitia of the aorta. Except in thin patients without retroperitoneal pathology, this is not always easy because the great vessels are covered by node-bearing tissue and cannot be seen. The level of the aortic bifurcation above the sacrum is also very variable. There are no certain landmarks other than the root of the mesentery which is elevated to retract the bowel. Palpating the sacrum and "feeling" the pulsations of the aorta with a dissecting probe may be helpful. However, this is not as clear as one might imagine.

It is much safer to incise the nodal tissue higher than lower because there are no important structures in front of the aorta below the root of the mesentery, except for the inferior mesenteric artery. The artery usually lies lateral to the aorta. If the dissection is started too low there is a danger of injuring the left common iliac vein below the bifurcation of the aorta. Once the plane between the aorta and the overlying nodal tissue has been developed and the glistening surface of the aorta is seen, the dissection is very straightforward. The only real challenge is to keep bowel out of the way. This is done by elevating the posterior parietal peritoneum.

The limits of the dissection are the aortic bifurcation inferiorly, and the proximal part of the common iliac artery infero-laterally. On the right the dissection is continued across the front of the vena cava until its lateral border is freed. On the left, the plane of dissection is underneath the inferior mesenteric artery distally, and then above the artery more proximally.

Although the feasibility of the left-sided dissection has been questioned by some oncologists, it is in fact safer, and no more difficult than the right side. However, the inferior mesenteric artery has to be dissected free. The superior limit of the dissection is the third part of the duodenum. It is a simple matter to mobilize the duodenum and expose the left renal vein (Fig. 16.6), but this is only necessary in cervical cancer if obvious lymph nodes are present in this area.

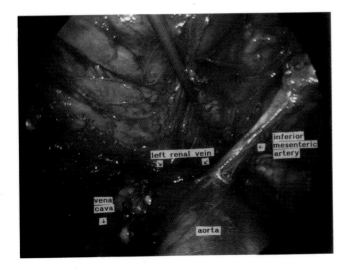

Figure 16.6 *Supramesenteric aortic lymphadenectomy.*

SUGGESTED READING

Childers JA, Surwit EA: Current status of operative laparoscopy in gynecologic oncology. *Oncology* 1993 **7**:47–51.

Kadar N: Laparoscopic pelvic lymphadenectomy for the treatment of gynecological malignancies: description of a technique. *Gynaecol Endosc* 1992 **1**:79–83.

Kadar N: Laparoscopic resection of fixed and enlarged aortic lymph nodes in patients with advanced cervix cancer. *Gynaecol Endosc* 1993 **2**:217–221.

Kadar N: An operative technique for laparoscopic radical vaginal hysterectomy and its evolution. *Gynaecol Endosc* 1994 **3**:69–74.

Kadar N, Pelosi MA: Can cervix cancer be adequately staged by laparoscopic aortic lymphadenectomy? *Gynaecol Oncol* (in press).

Kadar N, Reich H: Laparoscopically assisted radical Schauta hysterectomy and bilateral pelvic lymphadenectomy for the treatment of bulky stage IB carcinoma of the cervix. *Gynaecol Endosc* 1993 **2**:135–142.

Querleu D, Leblanc E, Castelain B: Laparoscopic lymphadenectomy in the staging of early carcinoma of the cervix. *Am J Obstet Gynecol* 1991 **164**:579–581.

17 LAPAROSCOPIC IDENTIFICATION OF THE URETER

Nicholas Kadar and Harry Reich

The standard method used to identify the ureter at laparotomy consists of blunt dissection medial to the hypogastric artery to open the para-rectal space where the ureter lies. This is very straightforward because once the broad ligament is opened, the bifurcation of the common iliac artery and the hypogastric artery can be easily identified by palpation. Unfortunately, this technique does not lend itself to a laparoscopic approach. First, with each step of the dissection, the tissue becomes progressively more slack, increasingly more difficult to put on tension, and eventually often impossible to dissect. This tends to occur if the round and infundibulo-pelvic ligaments are divided at the beginning of the dissection. Second, the hypogastric arteries are covered by lymph-bearing fatty-areolar tissue and cannot be visualized by merely opening the broad ligament, except in the thinnest of patients, and obviously cannot be palpated.

ANATOMY OF THE URETER

Approximately half way between the pelvic inlet and the renal pelvis the ovarian vessels cross the abdominal ureters to lie lateral to them at the pelvic brim (Fig. 17.1). Here, the ovarian vessels enter the infundibulo-pelvic ligament, cross the ureters again to lie at first above, and then medial to them, as the vessels run medially in the roof of the broad ligament to the ovaries and then the uterus. The surgi-cal significance of this relationship is that: (1) the ureter cannot be damaged if the pelvic sidewall peritoneum is incised lateral to the anatomic position of the infundibulo-pelvic ligament, and (2) the infundibulo-pelvic ligament can be retracted medially to expose the ureter at the pelvic brim and on the medial leaf of the broad ligament.

Throughout their pelvic course the ureters lie in a connective tissue sheath attached to the medial leaf of the broad ligament. After crossing the pelvic brim, the ureters follow the contours of the pelvis, and descend abruptly and laterally to run along the pelvic sidewalls just above the internal iliac arteries (Fig. 17.2). The left ureter is often found in a lower position than the right. These relations explain why it is frequently impossible to visualize the ureter by simply opening the broad ligament.

As the broad ligament is opened, the ureter will be displaced with its medial leaf to a position directly below the infundibulo-pelvic ligament, which runs in the roof of the broad ligament, and which will now cover the ureter. Distal to the pelvic brim, the ureter also lies quite deep in the pelvis further hidden from view by its covering of loose fatty-areolar tissue. If the round and/or infundibulo-pelvic ligaments are also divided at the beginning of the dissection, the tissue laxity created compounds these problems further rendering ureteric identification virtually impossible.

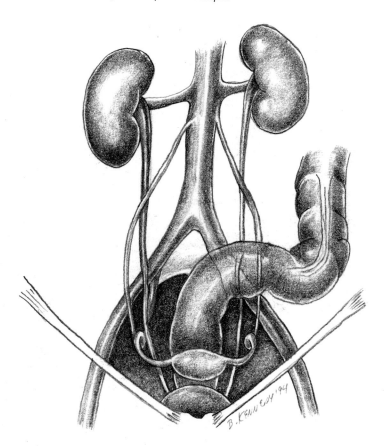

Figure 17.1 Relationship between the ureter and the ovarian vessels in the abdomen and pelvis. *From Kadar N:* Atlas of Laparoscopic Pelvic Surgery, *Blackwell Scientific Publications, Oxford, 1994.*

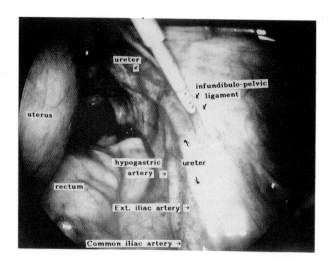

Figure 17.2 The anatomic position of the ureter as seen laparoscopically. *From Kadar N:* Atlas of Laparoscopic Pelvic Surgery, *Blackwell Scientific Publications, Oxford, 1994. Reproduced with permission.*

LAPAROSCOPIC TECHNIQUES TO IDENTIFY THE URETER

Three approaches have been used for laparoscopic ureteric identification, which may be called medial, superior and lateral. The lateral approach is the most versatile because, like its open counterpart, it makes use of the retroperitoneal spaces, which are opened in the process.

The medial approach

If the uterus is anteflexed, the ureter can usually be easily visualized in its natural position on the medial leaf of the broad ligament (at least on the right side) provided there is no significant cul de sac or adnexal pathology (Fig. 17.2). This allows the peritoneum immediately above the ureter to be incised to create a "window" in the peritoneum, which makes for safe division of the infundibulo-pelvic ligament or adnexal pedicle. The peritoneal incision must be very superficial, however; otherwise the iliac vessels which lie just lateral, out of view, can be injured.

This approach was popularized for laparoscopic hysterectomies by Reich, who feels that ureteral isolation should be an integral part of this procedure. Immediately after exploration of the upper abdomen and pelvis, each ureter is isolated deep in the pelvis, if possible. This is done early in the operation before the pelvic sidewall peritoneum becomes oedematous and/or opaque from irritation by the CO_2 pneumoperitoneum or aquadissection and before ureteral peristalsis is inhibited by surgical stress, pressure, or the Trendelenburg position. The left ureter is dissected first as it is usually more difficult to find. The ureter and its overlying peritoneum are grasped deep in the pelvis on the left below the lateral rectosigmoid attachments at the pelvic brim (Fig. 17.3) Atraumatic grasping forceps are used from a right-sided cannula to grasp the ureter and its overlying peritoneum on the left pelvic sidewall below and caudad to the left ovary, lateral to the left uterosacral ligament. Scissors are used to divide the peritoneum overlying the ureter and are inserted into the defect created and spread. Thereafter one blade of the scissors is placed on top of the ureter, the buried scissor blade visualized through the peritoneum, and the peritoneum divided. This is continued into the deep pelvis where the uterine vessels cross the ureter, lateral to the cardinal ligament insertion into the cervix. Connective tissue between the ureter and the vessels is separated with scissors (Fig. 17.4). Bleeding is controlled with microbipolar forceps. Often the uterine artery is ligated at this time to diminish backbleeding from the upper pedicles (Fig. 17.5). The procedure is repeated on the right side.

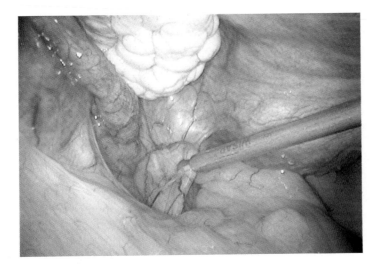

Figure 17.3 *Left ureter is grasped from right side. Peritoneum lateral to left ureter is then opened with laparoscopic scissors.*

This approach has not been duplicated by many other surgeons, who limit its usage to easy laparoscopic hysterectomies that many accomplished surgeons do vaginally. First, the left ureter frequently cannot be visualized in this way. Second, the technique obviously cannot be applied when there is significant pathology in the cul de sac or adnexa. Third, it does not allow proper access to the retroperitoneum and the development of the para-rectal space.

The superior approach

The superior approach entails dissecting the rectosigmoid off the left side of the pelvic brim and freeing the infundibulo-pelvic ligament vessels from the roof of the broad ligament. This allows the ureter that lies below it and the superior rectal artery to be identified. The ureter is then reflected off the broad ligament and traced into the pelvis. This approach has been replaced by the lateral approach, especially for difficult hysterectomies with matted down adnexa and radical pelvic surgery, allowing a more systematic development of the retroperitoneum.

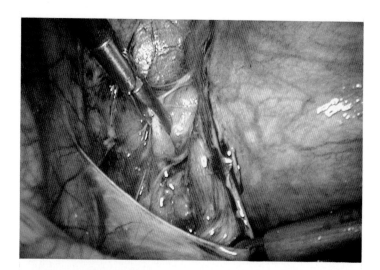

Figure 17.4 *Grasping forceps are used to separate left ureter from left uterine artery.*

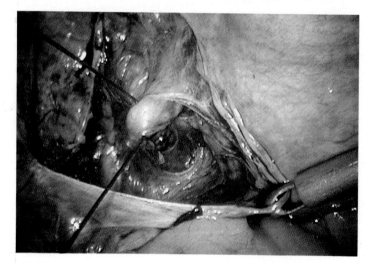

Figure 17.5 *Suture is applied around the left uterine artery.*

The lateral approach

The lateral approach is the laparoscopic equivalent of the open technique for it makes use of the para-rectal space to identify the ureter, and the ureter does not have to be peeled off the broad ligament for its entire pelvic course to be visible. The technique makes use of three basic strategies:

1. The sidewall peritoneum is incised without dividing the round ligament, and the infundibulo-pelvic or adnexal pedicles are only divided after the retroperitoneal dissection is complete.
2. The ureter is identified at the pelvic brim, before it dives deep into the pelvis; the infundibulo-pelvic ligament must be adequately mobilized to make this possible.
3. The obliterated hypogastric artery, which is easily identified and dissected free laparoscopically, is traced retrogradely to the origin of the uterine artery. The uterine artery, which runs on top of the cardinal ligament, marking the caudal (distal) border of the para-rectal space, is used as a landmark for the para-rectal space.

OPERATIVE TECHNIQUE

Step 1. The pelvic sidewall triangles are opened

The triangle of the pelvic sidewall is delineated by displacing the uterus to the contra-lateral side. The base of this triangle is formed by the round ligament, the lateral border by the external iliac artery, the medial border by the infundibulo-pelvic ligament, and the apex by where the infundibulo-pelvic ligament crosses the common iliac artery (Fig. 17.6). The peritoneum in the middle of the triangle is incised with dissecting scissors and the broad ligament opened by bluntly separating the extraperitoneal areolar tissues. Even tiny vessels should be coagulated because the slightest amount of bleeding can stain the extraperitoneal areolar tissues and obscure the view of the underlying structures.

The peritoneal incision is extended first to the round ligament, which is not divided at this time, and then to the apex of the triangle, lateral to the infundibulo-pelvic ligament (Fig. 17.7). It is important not to displace the infundibulo-pelvic ligament from its anatomic position before the peritoneal incision is completed. Otherwise the natural anatomic relationship between the ligament and ureter will be lost.

On the left side, so-called congenital adhesions attach the recto-sigmoid to the peritoneum laterally, at or just above the pelvic brim. These usually cover the apex of the pelvic triangle. The dissection on the left side is begun by separating these adhesions from the underlying peritoneum, and the pelvic sidewall triangle is opened at or near its apex (Fig. 17.8). (The external iliac artery will be

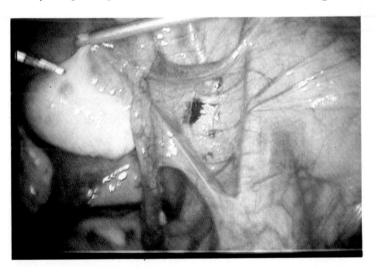

Figure 17.6 *The triangle of the pelvic sidewall is formed by the round ligament, the lateral border by the external iliac artery and the medial border by the infundibulo-pelvic ligament. From Kadar N:* Atlas of Laparoscopic Pelvic Surgery, *Blackwell Scientific Publications, Oxford, 1994. Reproduced with permission.*

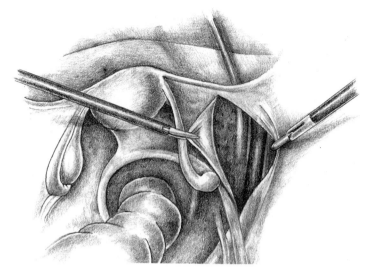

Figure 17.7 The peritoneal incision is extended to the round ligament and then to the apex of the triangle lateral to the infundibulo-pelvic ligament.
From Kadar N: Atlas of Laparoscopic Pelvic Surgery, *Blackwell Scientific Publications, Oxford, 1994.*

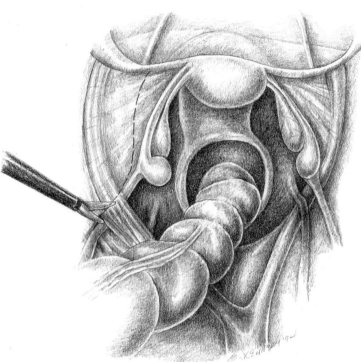

Figure 17.8 The attachments of the sigmoid colon are divided and the incision on the left is started at the apex of the pelvic sidewall triangle.
From Kadar N: Atlas of Laparoscopic Pelvic Surgery, *Blackwell Scientific Publications, Oxford, 1994.*

below the plane of dissection.) The peritoneal incision is then carried distally to the round ligament, which is again not divided at this time.

Step 2. The ureter is identified at the apex of the pelvic triangle

The infundibulo-pelvic ligament is pulled medially with grasping forceps to expose the ureter at the pelvic brim where it crosses the common or external iliac artery (Fig. 17.9). This is a crucial step. It may be necessary to reflect the ureter off the medial leaf of the broad ligament for a short distance to aid in its identification, although this is not always required.

It is important to mobilize the infundibulo-pelvic ligament adequately; otherwise it will not be possible to retract its proximal end

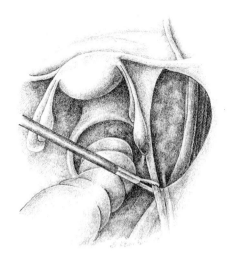

Figure 17.9 *The infundibulo-pelvic ligament is mobilized and pulled medially to expose the ureter at the pelvic brim.*
From Kadar N: Atlas of Laparoscopic Pelvic Surgery, *Blackwell Scientific Publications, Oxford, 1994.*

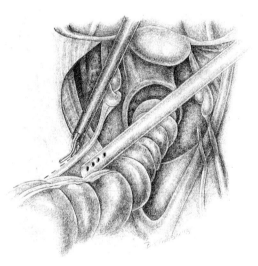

Figure 17.10 *Mobilization of the left infundibulo-pelvic ligament From Kadar N:* Atlas of Laparoscopic Pelvic Surgery, *Blackwell Scientific Publications, Oxford, 1994.*

sufficiently medially to expose the ureter at the pelvic brim. To achieve adequate mobilization, the peritoneal incision has to be extended much further proximally than in an open case, frequently to the caecum on the right, and the descending colon in the paracolic gutter on the left. Failure to achieve adequate mobilization of the infundibulo-pelvic ligament is the most common error in carrying out the dissection. The operator then searches for the ureter distal to the pelvic brim and lateral to the infundibulo-pelvic ligament, but frequently fails to find it for the ureter is at that point covered by fatty-areolar tissue, or, more distally, by the infundibulo-pelvic ligament itself, and cannot be seen except in the thinnest of patients.

The dissection of the apex is more difficult on the left side partly because the ureter is covered by the mesentery of the sigmoid colon, but mainly because it crosses the iliac vessels higher (more proximally), and consequently lies more medial than the right ureter. The peritoneal incision has to be extended to the white line in the paracolic gutter to mobilize the sigmoid colon, and with it the infundibulo-pelvic ligament, which at this point lie extraperitoneally, under the mesentery (Fig. 17.10). It may also be necessary to mobilize the medial leaf of the broad ligament from the pelvic brim and sacrum. To do this, the operator has to dissect bluntly in a medial direction under the infundibulo-pelvic ligament, taking care not to perforate the medial leaf of the broad ligament or the right plane of dissection will be lost. Finally, the operator needs to be aware that the external iliac artery will be below the plane of his dissection much of the time.

Step 3. The obliterated hypogastric arteries are identified extraperitoneally

The dissection is carried bluntly underneath and caudad to the round ligament, until the obliterated hypogastric artery is identified extraperitoneally (Fig. 17.11). Although the anatomy will be unfamiliar to most general

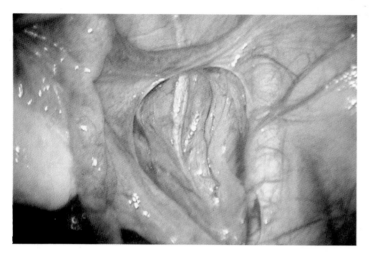

Figure 17.11 *The extraperitoneal portion of the obliterated hypogastric artery is identified. From Kadar N:* Atlas of Laparoscopic Pelvic Surgery, *Blackwell Scientific Publications, Oxford, 1994. Reproduced with permission.*

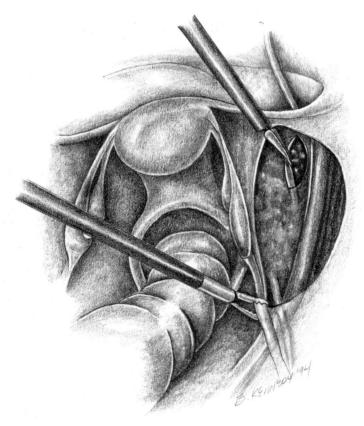

Figure 17.12 *The lateral para-vesical space is opened. From Kadar N:* Atlas of Laparoscopic Pelvic Surgery, *Blackwell Scientific Publications, Oxford, 1994.*

gynaecologists, this step is in fact the most straightforward part of the dissection. If any difficulty is encountered, the artery should be first identified intraperitoneally where it hangs from the anterior abdominal wall, traced proximally to where it passes behind the round ligament, and then with both its intraperitoneal portion and the dissected space under the round ligament in view, the intraperitoneal part of the ligament should be moved back and forth. It is usually possible to detect the corresponding movements in the extraperitoneal portion of the ligament.

Step 4. The para-vesical spaces are developed

Once the obliterated hypogastric arteries have been identified extraperitoneally it is a simple matter to develop the para-vesical space by bluntly separating the areolar tissue on either side of the artery. The dissection is started lateral to the artery, mindful that the external iliac vein is just lateral to it. The tips of the closed dissecting scissors are placed against the lateral edge of the artery and the artery is simply pulled medially, whereupon a bloodless plane will open lateral to it (Fig. 17.12).

The medial border of the artery is then freed in an identical manner, but working in the opposite direction. During this manoeuvre the operator must take care not to press on the external iliac vein as the artery is displaced laterally (Fig. 17.13).

Development of the para-vesical space is usually not required to resect residual ovaries or adnexal masses, but if a hysterectomy (simple or radical) and/or pelvic lymphadenectomy is to be carried out, they should be developed adequately to obtain good exposure of the uterine arteries and cardinal ligaments distally. This provides complete control of the operative field, especially if the arteries bleed when they are divided, which can occur despite what appears to be adequate bipolar desiccation.

Step 5. The para-rectal spaces are developed

The obliterated hypogastric arteries are next traced proximally to where they are joined by the uterine arteries, and the para-rectal spaces opened by blunt dissection proximal and medial to the uterine vessels, which lie on top of the cardinal ligaments. Once the para-rectal

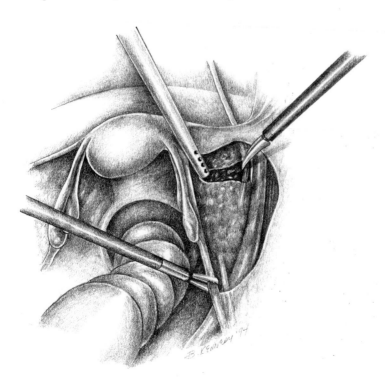

Figure 17.13 The medial para-vesical space is opened. From Kadar N: Atlas of Laparoscopic Pelvic Surgery, *Blackwell Scientific Publications, Oxford, 1994.*

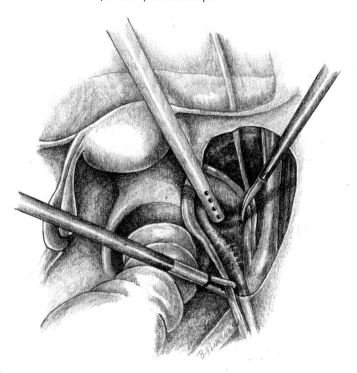

Figure 17.14 *The para-rectal space is developed; the ureter lies on its medial border.*

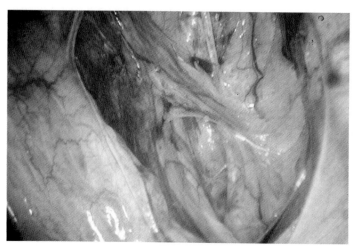

Figure 17.15 *All anatomical structures involved are demonstrated. Uterine artery is seen crossing right ureter after its origin from the hypogastric artery.*

spaces have been opened, the ureter on the ipsilateral side is easily identified on the medial leaf of the broad ligament, which forms the medial border of the para-rectal space. The uterine artery and cardinal ligament at the distal (caudal) border of the space, and the internal iliac artery on its lateral border also become clearly visible at this stage (Figs 17.14 and 17.15). The uterine artery can easily be ligated at this time.

SUGGESTED READING

Kadar N: *Atlas of Laparoscopic Pelvic Surgery.* Blackwell Scientific Publications, Boston, 1994, pp. 51–74.

Reich H: Pelvic sidewall dissection. In Hulka and Reich (eds) *Textbook of Laparoscopy,* 2nd Edn. WB Saunders, New York, 1994, p. 245.

18 LAPAROSCOPIC HYSTERECTOMY AND LAPAROSCOPIC ASSISTED VAGINAL HYSTERECTOMY

Liselotte Mettler and Kurt Semm

Laparoscopic assisted vaginal hysterectomy (LAVH) was initiated by Semm in 1982. The procedure was performed in women who have undergone many laparotomies, those who have severe intra-abdominal adhesions and in women with large benign ovarian cyst. The laparoscopic part was done to separate the adnexa from the pelvic wall and to dissect the mesosalpinx down to the cardinal ligaments. The dissection of the uterine vessels is done vaginally. In 1990, Reich reported LAVH with laparoscopic dissection of the ureters and uterine vessels and in 1991, Semm introduced classic intrafascial SEMM (serrated edged macro-morcellated) hysterectomy (CISH) without colpotomy.

Laparoscopic hysterectomy and LAVH have many advantages compared to an abdominal or pure vaginal hysterectomy. Blood loss is less, hospitalization time is shorter, the incidence of ileus is less and the risk of intra-abdominal adhesion formation is reduced. Furthermore, the pelvis can be thoroughly evaluated before uterine removal and adhesions, endometriosis or leiomyoma can be removed before the conduct of hysterectomy. In this chapter, we will describe several techniques of laparoscopic hysterectomy.

CLASSIC INTRAFASCIAL SUPRACERVICAL HYSTERECTOMY (CISH)

CISH was initiated by Semm as classic intrafascial SEMM (serrated edged macro-morcellated) hysterectomy. CISH can be done by laparoscopy, laparotomy or vaginally. The advantages of CISH are partial preservation of the integrity of the pelvic floor (no posterior colpotomy), preservation of blood supply to the pelvic floor, no interference with the sexual life and protection against cervical cancer by coring out the transformation zone. The estimated risk of cervical cancer following a supracervical hysterectomy is 0.3–0.9%. A modification of CISH is total uterine mucosa ablation (TUMA) where the residual uterine muscle remains *in situ*. This represents an alternative method to endometrial ablation.

The operating setup is depicted in Fig. 18.1. In CISH, there are two vaginal and two laparoscopy steps.

1. *First vaginal step*: The cervix is grasped with two tenaculae that are placed at the three and nine o'clock positions. Ten ml of 0.05% solution of vasopressin derivative (Rx POR-8, Ornipressin, Sandoz) is

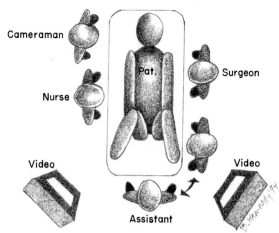

Figure 18.1 Operating theatre setup for the classic intrafascial supracervical hysterectomy (CISH).

injected into the cervix. The cervix–uterine length is measured and the cervix is dilated up to bougie Hegar #6. A calibrated uterine resection tool (CURT) to manipulate the uterus is introduced up to the uterine fundus (Figs 18.2A, 18.3 and 18.4). The tenaculae are attached to the guide rod by fixation screws.

2. *First laparoscopy step* (Fig. 18.2B–E): Adnexal dissection is done by applying sutures, suture ligatures or staples until the level of the cardinal ligaments (Fig. 18.2). After injection of POR-8 into the cervix, the bladder fold is dissected off the cervix with hook scissors and with a laparoscopic swab. A Roeder-loop is placed around the cervix and kept loose. The uterine vessels and ureters are not touched.

3. *Second vaginal step*: The CURT guide rod is perforated through the uterine fundus under laparoscopic control (Fig. 18.5). The inner layer of the cervix and uterus are carefully resected with the CURT by coring. The size of CURT is selected according to the measurement of the cervical diameter by ultrasound (10, 15, 20 or 24 mm). Coring is performed using a small battery device that automatically drives the coring device forward. As soon as the uterine fundus is perforated (Fig. 18.2E), the guide rod and the coring device are withdrawn and the Roeder-loop is tightened. This is to avoid loss of pneumoperitoneum. The resected uterine cylinder (Fig. 18.6) is sent for histopathological examination. The remaining cervical shell is endocoagulated with a haemostaser probe heated by an Erystop (Fig. 18.7). It is an endocoagulator with a coagulation power of 150 watts and a local heat production of 120°C. The tenaculae are released and the vaginal part is completed.

4. *Second laparoscopic step* (Figs 18.2F–I, 18.8 and 18.9): The tightened Roeder-loop is secured with a security knot and two more loops are placed, tightened and secured. The uterine corpus is grasped with a claw forceps and it is severed from the cervix with hook scissors. The cervical stump is disinfected with a disinfecting swab and endocoagulated. The cervical stump is then suspended to the round ligaments and the visceral peritoneum is closed over the cervix. The uterus is morcellated with serrated edged macro-morcellator (SEMM) and removed from the abdominal cavity. A drain tube is inserted via a 5-mm trocar and removed in 24 hours.

Figure 18.2 (opposite) *Steps for CISH:*

A. *Transcervical–transuterine perforation of the uterine fundus with the guide rod of the calibrated uterine resection tool (CURT).*

B. *Adnexal separation from the uterus after securing with suture–ligatures and extra-corporeal knot tying.*

C. *Infiltration of the cervix and the bladder fold with the vasopressin derivative POR-8.*

D. *Aquadissection and dissection of the bladder fold.*

E. *Placement of a Roeder-loop around the cervix and coring the transcervical–transuterine cylinder with the CURT.*

F. *Supracervical separation of the uterus with scissors.*

G. *Suspension of the cervical stump to the round ligaments bilaterally.*

H. *Peritoneal closure with a continuous suture.*

I. *Uterine morcellation with the serrated edged macro-morcellator (SEMM).*

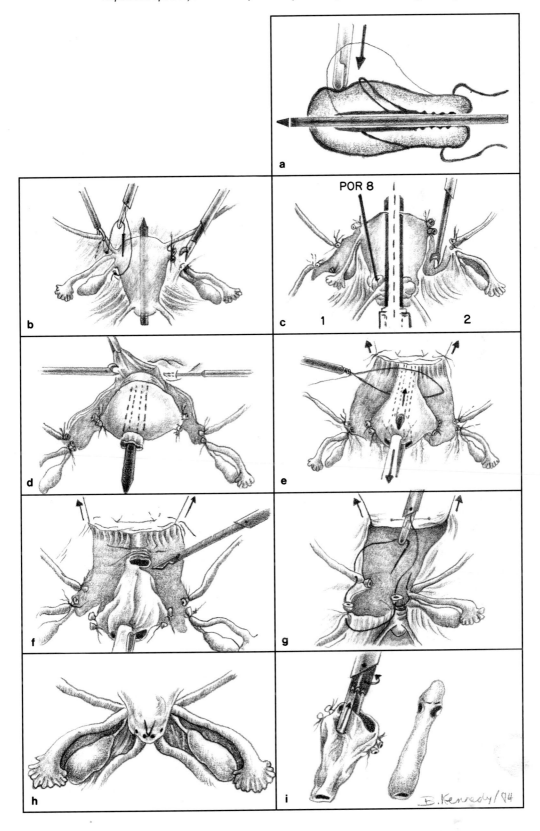

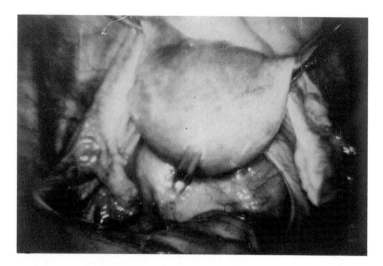

Figure 18.3 Placement of CURT guide rod through the uterine fundus.

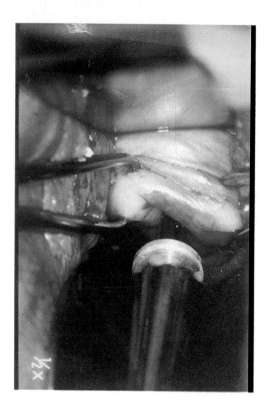

Figure 18.4 Cervical excoriation.

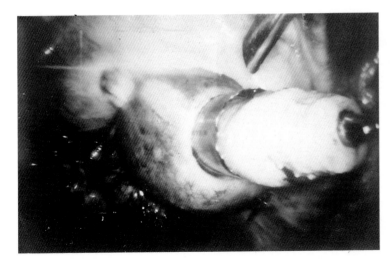

Figure 18.5 *Laparoscopic view of resection of the cervico-uterine mucosa.*

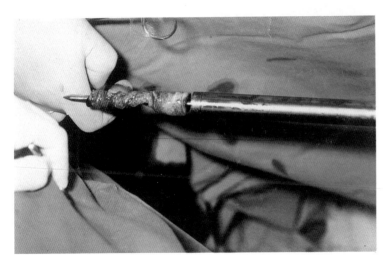

Figure 18.6 *Cervico-uterine cylinder.*

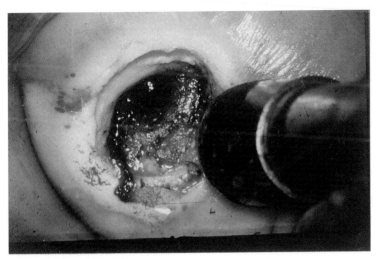

Figure 18.7 *Endocoagulation of the remaining part of the cervix with Erystop.*

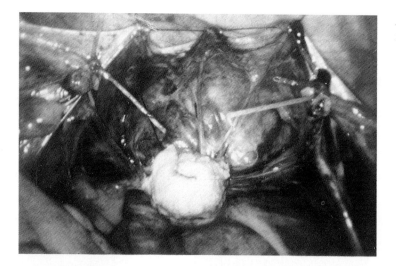

Figure 18.8 *Cervical stump after resection of the uterine corpus.*

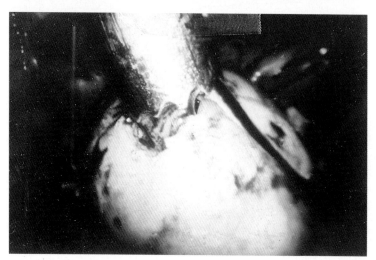

Figure 18.9 *Transabdominal morcellation of the uterus using the SEMM.*

Figure 18.10 (opposite) *Intrafascial vaginal hysterectomy (IVH).*   *a.* *Traction on cervix by two tenacula and opening of vaginal wall with scalpel from 9–3 o'clock (proximal to the vesico-uterine peritoneal fold). *b.* Measuring length of cervix and opening of peritoneum (colpotomia anterior). Dilatation of cervical canal Hegar 3–5.   *c.* Resetting of tenacula deep into parametria at 9 and 3 o'clock. Introduction of axial guide rod and CURT. Injection of 10 ml of 0.05 IU ml⁻¹ POR-8 or vasopressin solution on each side of cervix. *d.* Rotating cutting procedure manually or using WISAPᴿ-Moto-Drive. Required depth excoration 6–7 cm. Removal of CURT and guide rod.   *e.* Grasping excised cervical conus with claw forceps and removal of cervical muscle.   *f.* By rotating forceps, cervical and partly uterine muscle is removed like a myoma in status nascendi.   *g.* Closing excoriation wound with two temporary sutures. Anterior extraction of uterus with two catspaws. Adnexa either remain, are removed vaginally or, if indicated, are removed by pelviscopic assistance.   *h.* Vaginal grasping, ligation and transection of round ligaments. Setting ligature above cardinal ligaments and suture-ligation deep in excoriated cervix of ascending branches of uterine arteries on both sides. The ureters have been anteriorly displaced together with the bladder.   *i.* Supracervical resection of uterus using scalpel.   *j.* Suturing pedicles of round ligaments to pericervical tissue of cervical stump. At the end of the surgery the vesico-uterine peritoneum is sutured to the posterior wall of the cervical fascia, the vaginal wall wound is closed by interrupted sutures, the temporary sutures of the cervical excoriation wound are released and the cervical would can be coagulated.*

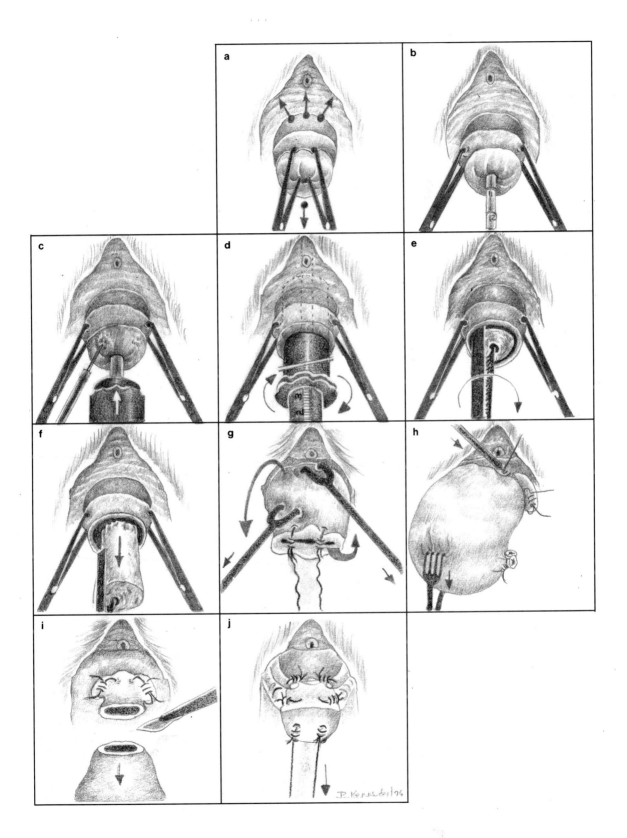

INTRAFASCIAL VAGINAL HYSTERECTOMY (IVH)

This is a modification of CISH where after punching out the cervical tissue, vaginal hysterectomy is performed in the usual manner. Here, the pelvic ligaments and vagina remain uninjured. (See Fig. 18.10.)

LAPAROSCOPIC ASSISTED VAGINAL HYSTERECTOMY (LAVH) AND TOTAL LAPAROSCOPIC ASSISTED VAGINAL HYSTERECTOMY (TLAVH)

One of the primary purposes of LAVH is to convert an abdominal hysterectomy to a vaginal procedure. Thus, essentially any condition that prevents a vaginal hysterectomy but can be solved laparoscopically represents an indication for LAVH. LAVH can be done with anterior or posterior colpotomy incision. The difference between LAVH and TLAVH is in the extent of laparoscopic dissection. In LAVH, the laparoscopic dissection along the cervix is stopped some distance above the uterine vessels. In TLAVH, dissection of the uterine vessels and the uterus is done laparoscopically and the vaginal part is done only to remove the uterus.

Laparoscopic assisted vaginal hysterectomy (LAVH)

LAVH (see Fig. 18.11) with anterior colpotomy is also called laparoscopic Döderlein hysterectomy. Haemostasis is done either with electrocautery, sutures, clips or staples. We use four trocars, a primary 10–12-mm trocar at the umbilical site, a 5-mm trocar at the midline two finger breadths above the symphysis pubis and two 10–12-mm trocars in the left and right low abdominal quadrant lateral to the rectus muscle. They are inserted at the level of the umbilicus if the uterus is large or 25 mm lower if the uterus is smaller than 12 weeks gestational size. The patient is placed in a deep Trendelenburg position without shoulder braces.

The course of the ureter should always be followed before and throughout the procedure. If the ovaries are to be removed, an Endo Gauge measuring instrument is placed on the infundibulo-pelvic ligament to determine the proper Multifire Endo GIA-30 cartridge for transecting the ligament. We usually place the Vascular Endo GIA stapler via the left lower quadrant port to transect the right infundibulo-pelvic ligament. Then, a second stapler is placed via the ipsilateral port to transect the broad and the round ligaments. If the ovaries are to be retained, transection is done on the utero-ovarian ligaments. First the camera is moved to the right lower quadrant port and the stapler is inserted through the 12 mm umbilical port. A second stapler is placed parallel to the uterine fundus incorporating the round ligament and the upper portion of the broad ligament.

The bladder flap is developed using sharp dissection with scissors. This can be facilitated by hydrodissection using solution of 0.05% POR-8. The bladder is dissected off the lower uterine segment and the cervix until the endopelvic fascia overlying the cervix is identified. This frequently requires the use of an endoscopic swab. Haemostasis, especially in the area of bladder pillar, should be secured. The course of the ureters is again followed. The last application of the stapler is on each side of the uterus parallel to the cervix stopping approximately 3 mm above the uterine artery. Note that the Multifire Endo GIA-30 spans 8 mm from the inside of the cartridge to

---

Figure 18.11 (opposite) *Laparoscopic assisted vaginal hysterectomy with bilateral salpingo-oophorectomy:*
1. Trocar sites. 2. Stapling the infundibulo-pelvic ligament. 3. Stapling the round ligament. 4. The development of the bladder flap. 5. Anterior colpotomy incision. 6. The fundus is delivered through an anterior colpotomy opening. 7, 8. Clamp, cut and suture–ligate the uterine vessels, cardinal ligaments and the uterosacral ligaments. 9. Clamp the posterior cuff, cut the specimen and suture the posterior cuff.

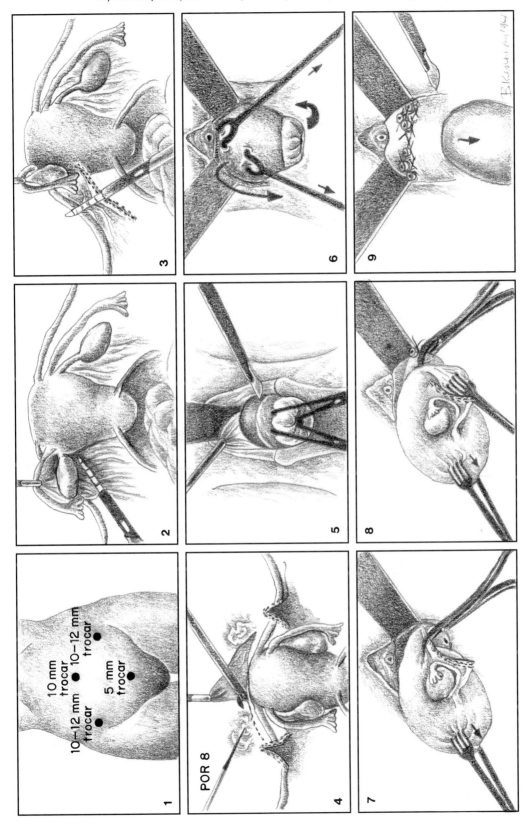

the outside row of staplers and often the space between the cervix and the ureter is less than 8 mm. Therefore, application of the stapler below the uterine vessels may be risky.

The vaginal portion of the procedure is depicted in Fig. 18.11. Note that the uterine fundus is delivered via an anterior colpotomy opening. This eliminates the necessity to perform a posterior colpotomy. The integrity of the posterior cul de sac is maintained and the risk of enterocele is reduced. After the vaginal cuff is closed, the operative field is inspected by laparoscope. This is done after the intra-abdominal pressure is decreased to 6 mmHg. Irrigation of the operative field and haemostasis are done if necessary.

Total laparoscopic assisted vaginal hysterectomy (TLAVH)

In TLAVH (see Fig. 18.12), the round ligament is divided using a stapler incorporating the posterior broad ligament. If the adnexa is to be removed, the incision is extended to the broad ligament lateral to the adnexa, lateral and parallel to the infundibulo-pelvic ligament. The infundibulo-pelvic ligament is then skeletonized, stapled and transected. If the ovary is to be preserved, the utero-ovarian ligament is transected. The ureters must always be identified and this can be achieved by opening the peritoneum above the pelvic brim or by dissecting the ureter on the pelvic sidewall. The bladder is then dissected off the cervix as in LAVH. In TLAVH, the uterine vessels are skeletonized, stapled and transected. Because of the close proximity of the vessels to the ureter, we recommend the use of mechanical devices such as stapler or clips. Skeletonization, stapling and transection are continued on the cardinal ligaments until the uterosacral ligaments. As in LAVH, in order to apply the stapler parallel to and adjacent to the uterus, the laparoscope must be placed in the lower trocar and the stapler in the umbilical port.

The colpotomy incision is then made. The site of colpotomy is determined with the help of vaginal and rectal probes. The remainder of the procedure is completed by the vaginal route. At the completion of the operation, all pedicles are inspected by the laparoscope to ascertain that haemostasis is secured.

POTENTIAL COMPLICATIONS AND THEIR PREVENTION

CISH and IVH involve excision of the functional tissue of the cervix. The risk of developing malignancy from the remaining cervical muscle and connective tissue is extremely small (1:100,000).

1. Pre-operative complication prevention. A pre-operative examination and possible bowel prep on the day prior to the operation are important. The availability of basic surgical instruments and apparatus including instruments for haemostasis such as clips, ligatures, sutures or staplers is mandatory. The patient is always prepared for a laparotomy in a way that a conversion to laparotomy is not considered a complication but an extension of the procedure for a better treatment.

2. Post-operative complication prevention. If adhesiolysis is performed, the patient should be warned about the symptoms of bowel perforation including pain, abdominal distention and ileus. Observations of post-operative fever, urinary symptoms, abdominal distention, bowel habit and abdominal pain are extremely important. If a drain is used, the colour and quantity of the drainage fluid should be evaluated.

3. A special risk of CISH is slippage of the loop around the cervical stump and bleeding from the ascending branch of the uterine arteries.

Figure 18.12 (opposite) *Total laparoscopic assisted vaginal hysterectomy (TLAVH) without salpingo-oophorectomy:*
1. Trocar sites. 2. Stapling the round ligament. 3. Stapling the infundibulo-pelvic ligament. 4. Injection of 10–20 ml of 0.05 IU ml⁻¹ POR-8 or vasopressin and development of bladder flap. 5. Stapling of cardinal ligament and uterine vessels – take care of ureters. 6. Stapling and transection of sacro-uterine ligaments. 7. Anterior and posterior colpotomy incisions. 8. Vaginal extraction of the uterus after cutting of remaining tissues.

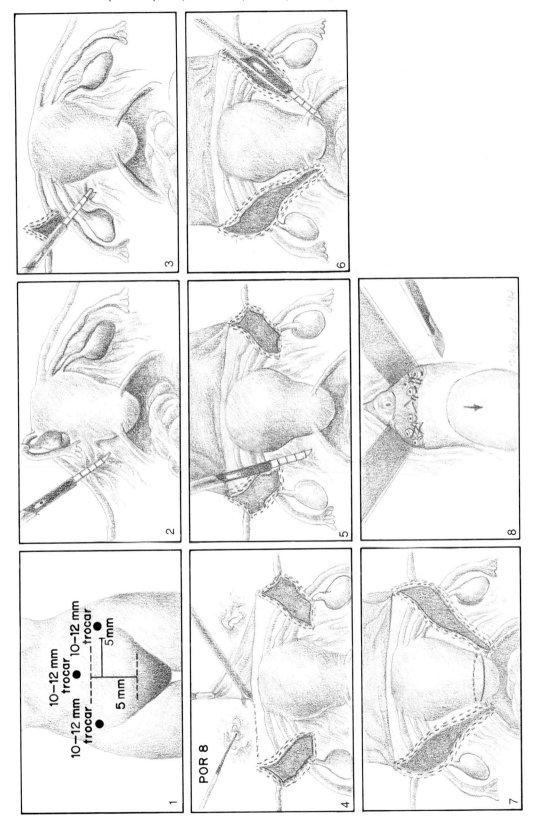

SUGGESTED READING

Mettler L: Einsatz des Endo-Staplers (Multifire Endo GIA™ 30) zur endosckopisscheen Ovar-, Adnex- oder Tubektomie sowie intrafaszialen Hysterektomie ohne Kolpotomie. *Minimal Invasive Chirurgie* 1993 **2**:10–13.

Mettler L, Semm K, Lüttges JE, Panadikar D: Pelviskopische intrafasziale hysterectomie ohne Kolpotomie (CISH). *Gynäkol Prax* 1993 **17**:509–526.

Nezhat CR, Burrell MO, Nezhat FR: Laparoscopic radical hysterectomy with paraaortic and pelvic node dissection. *Am J Obstet Gynecol* 1992 **166**:864–865.

Semm K: *Operationslehre für Endoskopische Abdominalchirurgie*. Schattauer, Stuttgart, 1984.

Semm K: Hysterektomie per laparotomiam oder per pelviscopiam. Ein neuer Weg ohne Kolpotomie durch CASH. *Geburtsh Frauenheilk* 1991 **51**:996–1003.

Semm K: Totale Uterus Mucosa Ablatio (TUMA)-CURT anstelle Endometrium-Ablation. *Geburtsh Frauenheilk* 1992 **52**:773–777.

19 BOWEL RESECTION RELATED TO ENDOMETRIOSIS

David B. Redwine

Laparoscopic bowel resection for endometriosis may be superficial, partial thickness, full thickness, or segmental. The lower colon is most frequently involved (Table 19.l). The main indication for bowel resection for endometriosis is for relief of symptoms which may be due to bowel disease. Pre-operative intestinal studies are usually negative because endometriosis rarely penetrates into the bowel lumen. If intestinal surgery is anticipated, a mechanical bowel prep is mandatory in case full-thickness penetration is necessary. While electrosurgical resection of intestinal lesions is possible in expert hands, sharp scissors, a grasper, and a needle driver will be the most useful tools for most surgeons. The surgeon must be expert in identification of all forms of endometriosis and must examine the frequently involved intestinal areas in all patients.

STAGES IN THE PROCEDURE

Superficial resection

The intraperitoneal colon has four layers: serosa, outer longitudinal muscularis, inner circular muscularis, and mucosa (Fig. 19.1a). The serosa is lost below the peritoneal reflection of the cul de sac. These layers can be used to the surgeon's tremendous advantage since they can be easily separated like peeling layers off an onion. Superficial lesions can be grasped and the scissors cut into the serosa and outer layer of muscularis adjacent to the lesion (Fig. 19.lb), working from several sides so that the lesion is surrounded by a line of incision. Otherwise the ease of dissection within the layers of the bowel wall may quickly lead the dissection past the lesion, leading to a larger than necessary defect. The defect in the bowel wall is closed with interrupted 3–0 silk suture (Fig. 19.1c).

Table 19.1 Anatomic sites of intestinal involvement by endometriosis among 353 patients with histologically proved intestinal endometriosis in the author's practice

Anatomic site	No. of patients
Sigmoid colon	234
Rectal nodule	155
Ileum	52
Appendix	33
Caecum	21

The sum of the number of patients exceeds 353 because some patients had more than one intestinal area involved by endometriosis.

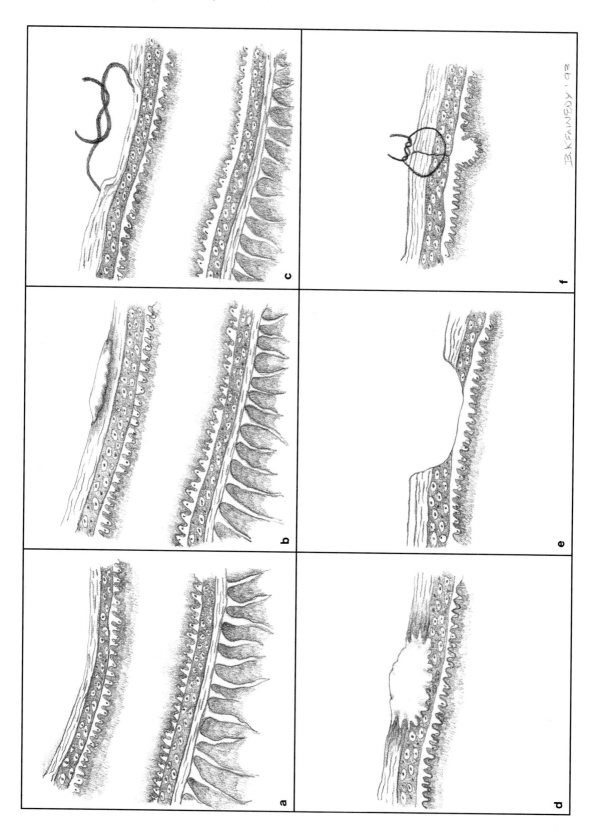

Mucosal skinning

Some larger invasive lesions involve both layers of muscularis (Fig. 19.1d). In such cases, the scissors cut through the normal bowel wall adjacent to the nodular invasive lesion until the dissection is sufficiently deep to undermine the lesion. The incision is made more or less perpendicularly into the bowel wall, working with a series of small cuts rather than one large cut. This way, the mucosa can squeeze out of the tips of the scissors, avoiding penetration into the lumen. Once the mucosa is encountered, the outer layers of muscularis containing the invasive lesion are now dissected bluntly off of the exposed mucosa (Figs 19.1e and 19.2). Once again, it is important to be aware of the linear extent of the lesion along the bowel wall, since it is easy to dissect far beyond. Several centimetres of mucosa can be exposed without entering the bowel lumen, allowing resection of large, bulky lesions. The seromuscular layers are closed with interrupted 3–0 silk sutures (Fig. 19.1f). Although there may be concern over inducing surgical distortion of the bowel wall by foreshortening the anterior bowel wall during suture closure, anterior muscularis defects up to 60 mm in length have been closed without producing symptoms of obstruction or obstipation.

Full-thickness resection

During mucosal skinning, it will become apparent that some invasive intestinal lesions extend to the submucosa. The resulting fibrosis can lead the dissection into the bowel lumen (Fig. 19.3). This allows direct palpation of the mucosa to determine where the submucosal fibrosis ends. The scissors cut into the mucosa around the nodularity, then back out through the bowel wall to the serosa. The mucosa is closed with running 3–0 chromic (Fig. 19.4) and the seromuscular layers are closed with interrupted 3–0 silk suture (Fig. 19.1f). Occasionally, a silk suture may penetrate the lumen without the surgeon's knowledge, but this is no cause for great concern since some bowel surgeons repair full thickness bowel injuries with a single layer of through-and-through interrupted silk sutures.

Obliteration of the cul de sac

When the rectosigmoid is adherent to the posterior cervix (Figs 19.5 and 19.6), such obliteration of the cul de sac usually signifies the presence of invasive disease of the uterosacral ligaments, cul de sac, and frequently the anterior rectal wall. Therefore, simply releasing the bowel from its adherence to the posterior cervix does nothing to treat invasive endometriosis. An *en bloc* resection of the pelvic floor combined with partial- or full-thickness bowel resection is necessary to ensure complete removal of all disease. The steps in treating obliteration of the cul de sac are consistently reproducible and represent largely an extension of resection of the uterosacral ligament described in Chapter 5 combined with the bowel resection techniques described above.

Releasing incisions are created in normal peritoneum lateral and parallel to the uterosacral ligaments (Fig. 19.7). This can

Figure 19.1 *(a) The anterior wall of the intraperitoneal colon is composed of four layers: serosa, outer longitudinal muscularis, inner circular muscularis, and mucosa. These layers can be peeled apart to the surgeon's advantage in treating colonic endometriosis. (b) Superficial lesions of endometriosis may involve only the serosa or outer longitudinal muscularis. (c) Superficial lesions can be removed by sharp excision into the outer longitudinal layer of muscularis, or into the inner circular muscularis. The defect is closed with interrupted 3–0 silk suture. (d) More invasive lesions of endometriosis may involve most of the inner circular muscularis. When submucosal fibrosis is absent, mucosal skinning may be used to remove such a lesion without penetration into the bowel lumen. (e) The involved layers of muscularis have been removed, with the mucosa exposed. (f) The seromuscular layer is closed with interrupted 3–0 silk sutures.*

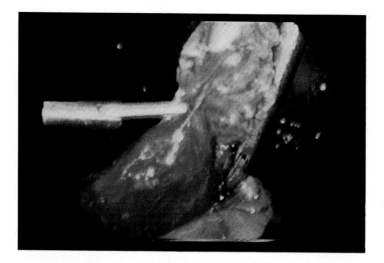

Figure 19.2 *The 3-mm scissors are bluntly dissecting both layers of colonic muscularis from the mucosa.*

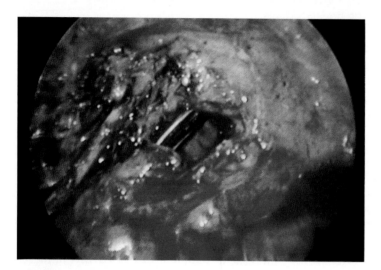

Figure 19.3 *Full-thickness bowel wall resection for excision of invasive intestinal endometriosis as viewed from a laparoscope inserted through a right lower quadrant port. The posterior cervix is out of the top of the frame. The shaft of a ring forceps passed through the anus can be seen traversing across the full-thickness defect in the bowel wall. Invasive endometriosis of the bowel is commonly associated with partial or complete obliteration of the cul de sac. Such cul de sac obliteration often is associated with retroperitoneal fibrosis which may involve the ureter. The left ureter is seen to the left of the rectosigmoid colon. It has been freed from retroperitoneal fibrosis by ureterolysis.*

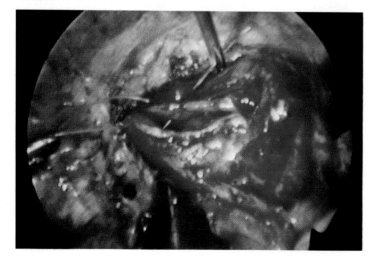

Figure 19.4 *Full-thickness bowel wall resection for excision of invasive intestinal endometriosis. The mucosa is being closed with running 3–0 chromic.*

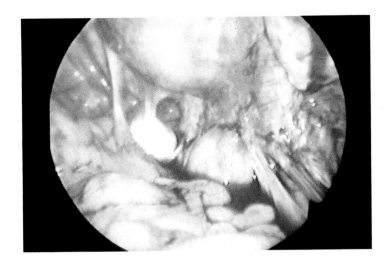

Figure 19.5 *Complete obliteration of the cul de sac. The uterine fundus is at the centre top of the frame. The left ovary is partially seen as a white ovoid object in the left centre of the frame. The right ovary is adjacent to the uterine fundus in the right upper quadrant of the frame. The rectosigmoid colon is adherent to the posterior cervix and both uterosacral ligaments. For successful treatment of this lesion, it must be assumed that invasive endometriosis involves the uterosacral ligaments, posterior cervix, cul de sac, and anterior bowel wall.*

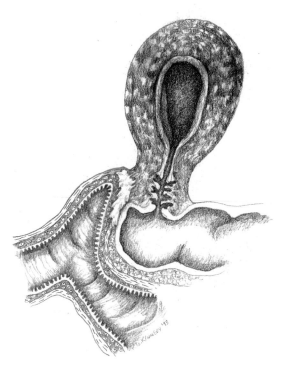

Figure 19.6 *Sagittal view of obliterated cul de sac. The invasive disease of the uterosacral ligaments is not shown in this view. The volume of invasive disease is therefore much larger than it appears in this representation. In some patients, the invasive disease may also invade the adjacent vaginal wall. In such cases, the dissection must enter the vagina immediately posterior to the cervix and exit the vagina into the rectovaginal septum distal to the involved vaginal mucosa.*

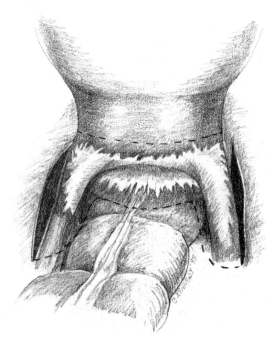

Figure 19.7 *Releasing incisions are made in the peritoneum lateral and parallel to the uterosacral ligaments. The dashed lines represent future lines of incision to be made across the posterior cervix and across the bowel wall. These incisions result in the progressive isolation of the invasive disease into the centre of the pelvis. Successful treatment of the obliterated cul de sac does not involve release of the obliteration.*

then be bluntly undermined. The ureter and uterine artery and vein are bluntly dissected laterally, and the peritoneal incision usually results in automatic separation of these vital structures from the uterosacral ligament. Another set of vessels courses up the postero-lateral vaginal wall, ascending just lateral to the uterosacral ligaments and anastomosing with the uterine artery and vein. It is important to anticipate these vessels to avoid injury to them. A transverse incision is made across the posterior cervix above the line of adherence of the colon (Fig. 19.8), and then an intrafascial dissection is carried down the posterior cervix toward the rectovaginal septum (Fig. 19.9). A layer of cervix approximately 2–4 mm in thickness is taken from the posterior body of the cervix (Fig. 19.10) in order to remove any invasive disease in this region. Occasionally the surgeon will see the release of small pockets of brownish fluid, indicating that invasive disease extends even deeper. In such cases, the dissection must proceed even deeper into the cervical stroma, although care must be taken to note entry into the cervical canal. If entry into the cervical canal occurs, it must be repaired in layers to avoid a cervico-peritoneal fistula.

Once the fatty tissue of the rectovaginal septum has been encountered (Fig. 19.11), the incisions lateral to the uterosacral ligaments are now carried around the posterior extent of invasive disease of these ligaments, then across the normal serosa of the anterior bowel wall proximal to the invasive lesion (Fig. 19.7). The obliterated cul de sac remains

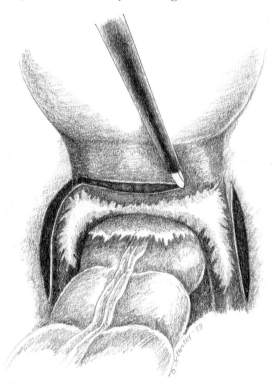

Figure 19.8 *The 3-mm monopolar scissors using 70 watts of cutting current or 50 watts of coagulation current are used to create a transverse incision across the posterior cervix above the adherent bowel. This incision will join the two peritoneal incisions lateral to the uterosacral ligaments.*

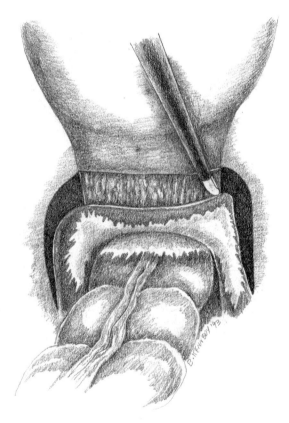

Figure 19.9 *This incision will be carried down the posterior cervix, removing a layer of cervical parenchyma approximately 2–3 mm thick so as to remove any invasive endometriosis in this area. The incision is directed posteriorly toward the rectovaginal septum, which will eventually be encountered.*

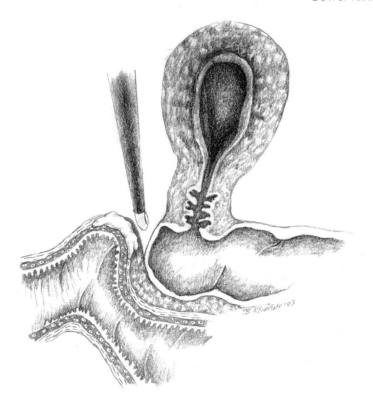

Figure 19.10 *A sagittal view of Fig. 19.9. A thin layer of posterior cervix has been removed and remains attached to the invasive endometriosis of the obliterated cul de sac and bowel wall. The rectovaginal septum is being approached.*

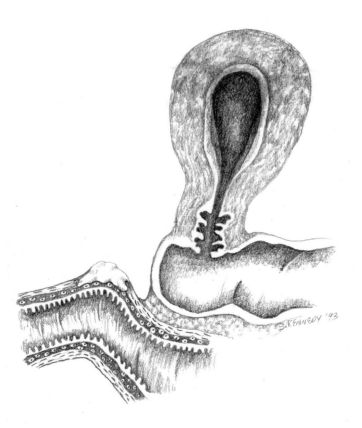

Figure 19.11 *Sagittal view. The rectovaginal septum has been encountered and the invasive endometriosis of the obliterated cul de sac has been mobilized into the anterior bowel wall. The uterosacral ligaments are not seen in this view but remain attached to this invasive nodule.*

obliterated, but it is now isolated in the centre of the pelvis attached to the anterior bowel wall. The lateral attachments of the recto-sigmoid are severed, thus restoring complete mobility to the involved segment of bowel (Fig. 19.12). The bulky nodular lesion (composed of the posterior cervix, uterosacral ligaments, obliterated cul de sac and anterior bowel wall) can now be removed from the bowel by superficial resection, mucosal skinning, or full-thickness resection with repair as discussed above (Figs 19.1–19.4). When full-thickness resection has occurred, the lesion can be removed transanally.

Segmental bowel resection

When a very large bowel nodule is present, or when several nodules are in close proximity, the defect in the anterior bowel wall resulting from local resection might be impossible to close primarily. In such rare cases, a laparoscopic segmental bowel resection with stapled anastomosis can be considered. Although this is technically feasible, its application would typically follow a potentially long and difficult pelvic dissection to remove all other pelvic disease and to free the involved bowel segment. Laparoscopic segmental bowel resection itself is a challenging procedure which may take several hours to accomplish. Most surgeons would serve their patients better by performing all laparoscopic surgery possible then opening the abdomen with a limited incision to complete the bowel resection (laparoscopically assisted bowel resection).

Resection of the ileum

The general principles of partial-thickness resection, mucosal skinning and full-thickness resection discussed above also apply to the ileum. Since the ileal wall is thinner than the colonic wall, full-thickness penetration during surgery is more likely. The mucosa can be closed with a separate suture of 3–0 chromic, and the seromuscularis with interrupted 3–0 silk.

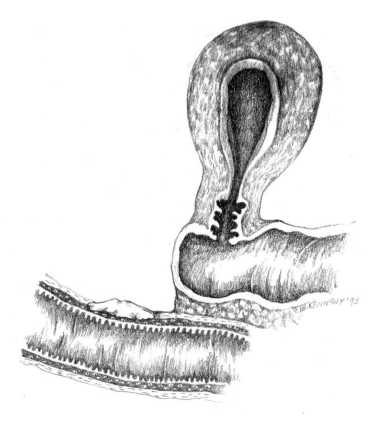

Figure 19.12 *The bowel has been completely mobilized. All invasive disease remains attached to the anterior bowel wall. The cul de sac remains obliterated. The uterosacral ligaments are not seen in this sagittal view.*

POTENTIAL COMPLICATIONS

Of 353 patients having biopsy-proven bowel endometriosis in the author's private practice, 148 have undergone laparoscopic treatment of bowel lesions, including 27 patients with full-thickness resections and three with segmental resections with end-to-end anastomosis. Two patients had an aborted laparoscopic segmental resection due to technical difficulty with the stapler and required a laparotomy to complete the procedure. Serious complications have been rare. One patient had a low-grade post-operative fever which responded to intravenous and oral antibiotics. Another undergoing a long (7 hours) procedure had bilateral peroneal nerve palsies which resolved spontaneously. Another undergoing partial-thickness resection without suture repair had late perforation of her sigmoid colon six days post-operatively which was repaired laparoscopically within 4 hours of occurrence with no further problems. A final patient with a prolonged bleeding time had a small painful pelvic haematoma which resolved after 10 days of observation.

CONTRAINDICATIONS

There are no specific medical contraindications to laparoscopic bowel resection if a patient is already to undergo laparoscopy. Lack of a bowel prep is a relative contraindication, since penetration of the unprepared bowel carries an increased risk of post-operative infection. However, in skilled hands, mucosal skinning can be performed safely without a bowel prep. Inexperience of the surgeon and inability to suture laparoscopically are other potential contraindications to laparoscopic bowel surgery.

SUGGESTED READING

Coronado C, Franklin RR, Lotze EC, Bailey HR, Valdes CT: Surgical treatment of symptomatic colorectal endometriosis. *Fertil Steril* 1990 **53**:411–416.

Nezhat F, Nezhat C, Pennington E: Laparoscopic proctectomy for infiltrating endometriosis of the rectum. *Fertil Steril* 1992 **57**:1129–1132.

Nezhat F, Nezhat C, Pennington E, Ambroze W: Laparoscopic segmental resection for infiltrating endometriosis of the rectosigmoid colon: a preliminary report. *Surg Laparosc Endosc* 1992 **2**:212–216.

Redwine DB, Sharpe DR: Laparoscopic segmental resection of the sigmoid colon for endometriosis. *J Laparoendoscopic Surg* 1991 **1**:217–220.

Redwine DB: Laparoscopic en bloc resection for treatment of the obliterated cul de sac in endometriosis. *J Reprod Med* 1992 **37**:695–698.

Redwine DB: Laparoscopic excision of endometriosis by sharp dissection. In Soderstrom RA (ed) *Operative Laparoscopy, The Masters' Techniques*. Raven Press, New York, 1993, pp. 101–106.

Reich H, McGlynn F, Salvat J: Laparoscopic treatment of cul-de-sac obliteration secondary to retrocervical deep fibrotic endometriosis. *J Reprod Med* 1991 **36**:516–522.

Sharpe DR, Redwine DB: Laparoscopic segmental resection of the sigmoid and rectosigmoid colon for endometriosis. *Surg Laparosc Endosc* 1992 **2**:120–124.

20 LAPAROSCOPIC TREATMENT OF URINARY STRESS INCONTINENCE

Thomas L. Lyons

Stress urinary incontinence (USI) is an endemic problem which impacts significantly on the patient's lifestyle and long-term psychological and physical health. Because medical therapy is successful in up to 70% of patients with USI, it should remain the standard treatment. However, in severe stress incontinence in conjunction with other associated gynaecological pathology, surgery may be indicated. Needle procedures (Raz, Perrer, Stamey, Gittes) and anterior colporrhaphy offer the lowest morbidity but are associated with the highest failure rates (up to 40–50%). Retropubic approaches (Marshall–Marchetti–Krantz, Burch) have become the surgery of choice with long-term success rates of 80–90%. However, these highly effective procedures require a large abdominal incision and they are usually reserved for patients who have failed vaginal surgery or are having other abdominal surgery. For this reason and with the conversion of many laparotomy procedures to laparoscopies, endoscopic or minimally invasive retropubic culposuspension (MIRC) is an excellent alternative. Furthermore, superior visualization is provided by laparoscopy. It can also be done in conjunction with other laparoscopic surgery including hysterectomy. Several techniques using sutures, staples or surgical mesh have been described.

PATIENT SELECTION

Patients selected for urethropexy should be carefully evaluated and should have genuine stress incontinence with or without associated detrusor symptomatology. The urethral sphincteric mechanism must be intact and urethral support (anterior vaginal wall mobility) must be defective. Other gynaecological problems, voiding habits, neurological symptoms, and current medication should be recorded. The symptoms of stress incontinence must be expressed by the patient and associated pelvic pathology should be noted. Neurologic assessment, urinalysis and urine culture, demonstration of the presence of stress incontinence and a Q-tip test should also be done. A timed void can be used to rule out decreased bladder capacity and voiding disorders. If a confusing clinical picture is presented, multichannel urodynamics and/or voiding cystometrics may be indicated. Patients with other medical conditions which would preclude surgery, patients who have not tried medical approaches, patients with voiding disorders or patients with a shortened or scarred anterior vaginal wall should be excluded from this procedure. Detrusor instability or previous surgery are not absolute contraindications for the procedure; in these cases pre-operative evaluation should be expanded.

PROCEDURE

The patient is consented for retropubic urethropexy with the possibility of laparotomy as for all laparoscopic procedures. Prophylactic antibiotics are given. A 30 cm³ Foley catheter inflated to 20 cm³ is used to assist in identification of the urethro-vesical (U/V) junction. Either of two approaches may be used to enter the space of Retzius. In the preperitoneal approach an open (Hasson) trocar is inserted at the umbilicus and CO_2 gas is insufflated into the preperitoneal space. The space is dissected by blunt dissection through the operating channel of the laparoscope. Once the space is opened a second 10–12-mm trocar is placed on the midline one to two finger breadths above the symphysis pubis. A 5-mm trocar is then placed lateral to the rectus muscle avoiding the epigastric vasculature. These trocars are inserted under laparoscopic control.

In the transperitoneal approach (usually dictated by other concomitant procedures), four trocars are placed in the standard manner. Two trocars of 10–12 mm are inserted at the subumbilical site and at the midline suprapubic site, and two trocars of 5 mm are inserted lateral to the right and left rectus muscles. The entry to the retroperitoneal space is made by incising the peritoneum 25 mm above the symphysis pubis transversely extending to the obliterated umbilical ligaments (Fig. 20.1). Blunt dissection is then carried out using an endoscopic Kittner over the operator's fingers which are placed in the vaginal vault to identify the fascia lateral to the U/V junction (Figs 20.2–20.4). Cooper's ligaments are also readily identified bilaterally. These structures are cleaned from excessive fat and areolar tissue. Figure-of-eight sutures using 0-Vicryl or 0-Ethibond on a CT-3 needle are then placed 10–20 mm lateral to the U/V junction bilaterally (Figs 20.5 and 20.6). The sutures are placed with the operator's fingers in the vagina to assist identification of the U/V junction. One of two techniques is then used. An endoknot loop can be stapled into Cooper's ligament with an endoscopic stapler (Fig. 20.7). As the loop is shortened the U/V angle is increased with elevation (the Nolan–Lyons modification, Figs 20.8 and 20.9). Alternatively, the figure-of-eight suture can be placed at the U/V angle and one arm of the suture is stapled to Cooper's ligament with an EMS stapler. The suture is tied extracorporeally. Additional sutures can then be placed to further lengthen the urethra and adequately elevate the U/V angle. After haemostasis is secured, all the instruments are removed and the incisional sites are closed. In the transperitoneal approach, the peritoneum is closed with a purse string suture. A posterior culdoplasty

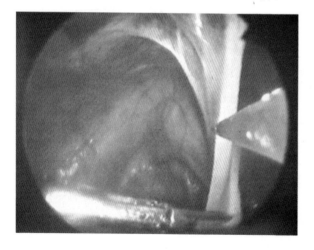

Figure 20.1 *Transperitoneal approach: opening the peritoneum 25 mm above the symphysis.*

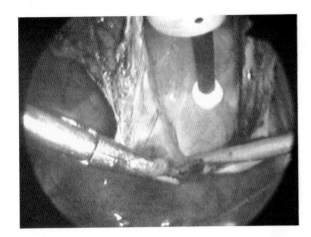

Figure 20.2 *Blunt dissection of the retropubic space using an endoscopic Kittner.*

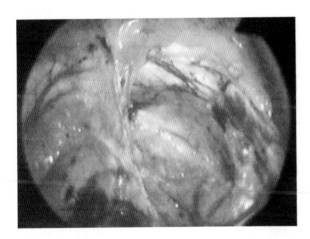

Figure 20.3 *Cooper's ligaments are exposed. The Foley bulb can be seen at six o'clock.*

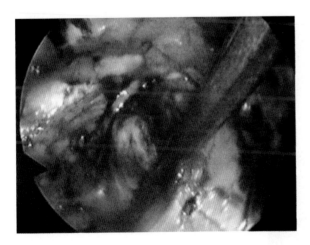

Figure 20.4 *An external view of the dissection of the paravaginal fascia with the operator's hand in the vagina. The corresponding Kittner dissection of U/V angle is shown.*

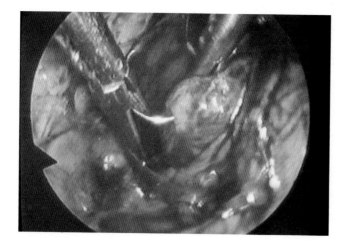

Figure 20.5 *Placement of the left U/V angle (paravaginal fascia) suture is seen. The CT-3 needle and suture has been back loaded.*

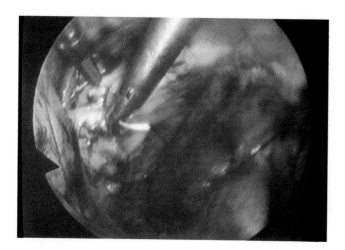

Figure 20.6 *The suture is passed through Cooper's ligament on the left side.*

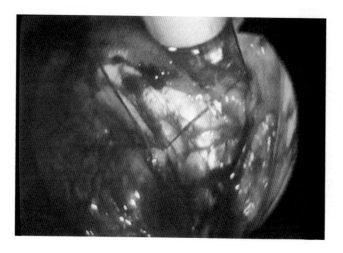

Figure 20.7 *The endoscopic stapler is used to secure one arm of the suture on the right side to Cooper's ligament.*

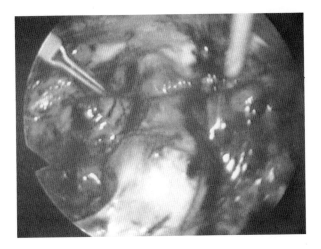

Figure 20.8 *The sling is clearly demonstrated with instruments over each of the Cooper's ligament attachments. The U/V angle and Foley bulb is seen at mid-picture.*

(Moschcowitz or Halban) is also performed to prevent enterocele in some patients. (A drain may be left in the space of Retzius if the operator desires.)

The Foley catheter is removed immediately after surgery and the patient is allowed to void. If difficulty in voiding is noted, the Foley catheter is reinserted and connected to a leg bag. It can be removed 24–48 hours later. Post-operative instructions include limitation of vigorous activity or straining for two weeks. The patient is allowed to resume normal activities immediately.

POTENTIAL COMPLICATIONS

Morbidity from the Burch procedure is usually associated with prolonged hospitalization and the length of catheterization. However, marked improvement has been seen with the laparoscopic approach. Because of the suturing aspects of the procedure, it is a technically demanding surgery, but patient performance to-date has been excellent. Injuries to bladder and urethra are commoner in patients who have had prior surgery in the space of Retzius. Bleeding and/or infection should remain minimal secondary to the minimally invasive approach.

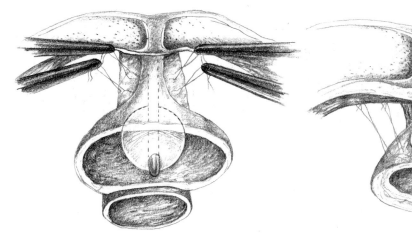

Figure 20.9 *Diagram of laparoscopic Burch procedure.*

Culposuspension can result in posterior defects (rectocule or enterocule) in a significant proportion of patients. Therefore, posterior supportive procedures should be accomplished during the surgery to prevent these problems, allowing a total approach to the pelvic floor.

Detrusor symptomology is common postoperatively but should resolve within 2 weeks. Post-operative patients with persistent symptoms can be treated medicinally with α-adrenergic agents or anticholinergic medications.

SUGGESTED READING

Burch JC: Urethrovaginal fixation to Cooper's ligament for correction of stress incontinence, cystocele and prolapse. *Am J Obstet Gynec* 1961 **81**:281.

Davis GD, Lobel RW: Laparoscopic retropubic colposuspension: the evolution of a new needle procedure. *Proceedings of World Congress of Gynecologic Endoscopy*, 22nd Annual Meeting of the American Association of Gynecology Laparoscopists, 1993.

Horbach NS: Genuine SUI: best surgical approach. *Contemp Obstet Gynecol* 1992, **37**, Special issue: Urogynecology.

Lie CY: Laparoscopic retropubic colposuspension (Burch procedure). *Gynecol Endo* 1993 **2**, No. 2.

Lyons TL: Minimally invasive retropubic urethropexy, the Nolan/Lyons modification of the Burch procedure. *Proceedings of World Congress of Gynecologic Endoscopy*, 22nd Annual Meeting of the American Association of Gynecology Laparoscopists, 1993.

Marshall VF, Marchetti AA, Krantz KE: The correction of stress incontinence by simple vesicourethral suspension. *Surg Gynecol Obstet* 1949 **88**:590.

Ou CS, Presthus J, Beadle E: Laparoscopic bladder neck suspension using hernia mesh. *Proceedings of World Congress of Gynecologic Endoscopy*, 22nd Annual Meeting of the American Association of Gynecology Laparoscopists, 1993.

Vancaillie TG, Schuessler W: Laparoscopic bladder neck suspension. *J LapEndo Surgery* 1991 **1**, No. 3.

21 APPENDECTOMY

Togas Tulandi

Routine incidental appendectomy at the time of other abdominal or gynaecological operations has been shown to be safe without an increase in morbidity. The implications of its conduct during a reproductive surgery remain unclear. However, if during a laparoscopy examination, an inflamed appendix or appendiceal endometriosis is found, an appendectomy should be done.

The appendix is grasped with grasping forceps and gently stretched. If adhesion is encountered, this has to be dissected first. Using a bipolar cautery, the mesoappendix is coagulated approximately 10 mm beyond the base of the appendix (Fig. 21.1) and then divided (Fig. 21.2). Alternatively, the appendiceal vessels can be secured with staples.

A pretied ligature (Endoloops, Rx Ethicon Inc., Sommerville, NJ; PercLoop, Laparomed, Irvine, CA) is applied around the base of the appendix, tightened and cut (Figs 21.3 and 21.4). A second ligature is placed close and distal to the first and a third ligature is placed approximately 10 mm from the second. The appendix is transected between the second

Figure 21.1

Figures 21.1 and 21.2 *Coagulation and cutting of mesoappendix approximately 10 mm beyond the base of the appendix.*

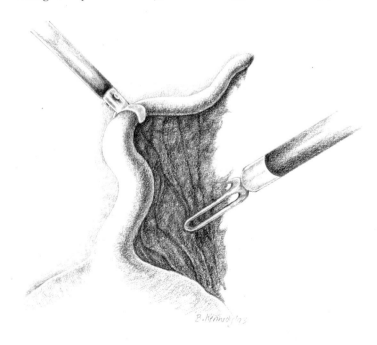

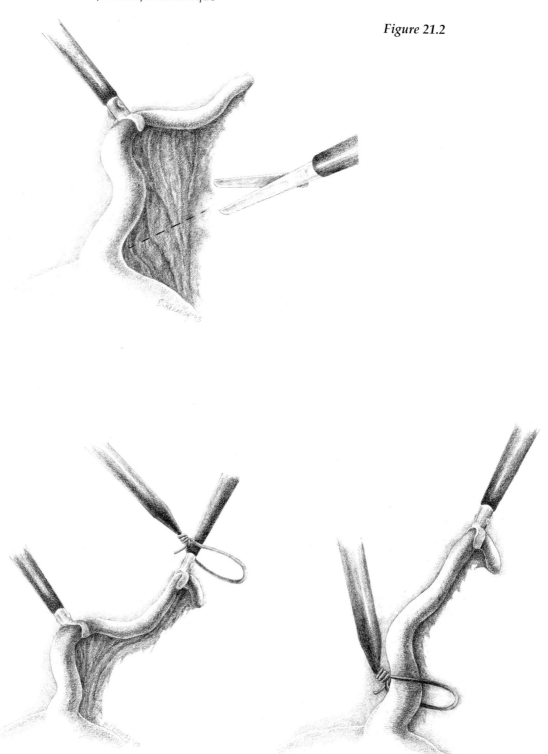

Figure 21.2

Figure 21.3

Figure 21.4

Figures 21.3 and 21.4 *Placement of a pretied ligature.*

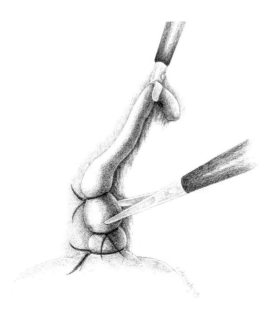

Figure 21.5a
Figures 21.5a and 21.5b Transection of the
appendix between the second and the third ligatures.

Figure 21.5b

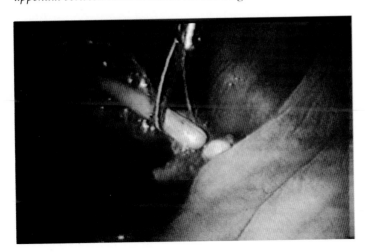

and the third loop (Fig. 21.5) and then
removed from the abdominal cavity via a
12 mm portal. The appendiceal stump is
coagulated lightly with bipolar coagulation or
vaporized with a laser.

POTENTIAL COMPLICATIONS AND THEIR PREVENTION

1. Leakage from the stump: make sure that
   the loops are tight.
2. Bleeding: good haemostasis.
3. Caecal perforation due to heat damage.
4. Abscess.

CONTRAINDICATIONS

Contraindications to appendectomy include patients who are unstable, patients with Crohn's disease and patients undergoing radiotherapy. Retrocaecal and a walled-off perforated appendix is also better approached by laparotomy.

SUGGESTED READING

Pier A, Gotz F, Bacher C, Thevissen P: Laparoscopic appendectomy in 625 cases: from innovation to routine. *Surg Laparosc Endosc* 1991 **1(1):** 8–13.

Richards W, Watson D, Lynch G, Reed GW, Olsen D, Spaw A, Holcomb W, Frexes-Steed M, Goldstein R, Sharp K: A review of the results of laparoscopic versus open appendectomy. *Surg Gynecol Obstet* 1993 **177:**473–480

SUBJECT INDEX